This is Our Child

How Parents Experience the Medical World

Edited by

ANTONYA COOPER

and

VALERIE HARPIN

Oxford   New York   Tokyo

OXFORD UNIVERSITY PRESS

1991

Oxford University Press, Walton Street, Oxford OX2 6DP

Oxford New York Toronto
Delhi Bombay Calcutta Madras Karachi
Petaling Jaya Singapore Hong Kong Tokyo
Nairobi Dar es Salaam Cape Town
Melbourne Auckland

and associated companies in
Berlin Ibadan

Oxford is a trade mark of Oxford University Press

Published in the United States
by Oxford University Press, New York

British Library Cataloguing in Publication Data
This is our child : how parents experience the medical
world. – (Oxford paperbacks).
1. Paediatrics. Social aspects
I. Cooper, Antonya II. Harpin, Valerie
362. 19892
ISBN 0-19-261899-7

Library of Congress Cataloging in Publication Data
Cooper, Antonya.
How parents experience the medical world / Antonya Cooper, Valerie
Harpin.
1. Sick children–Psychology–Case studies. 2. Sick children–Family relationships–Case
studies. 3. Children–Death–Psychological aspects–Case studies. 4. Adjustment
(Psychology)–Case studies. I. Harpin, Valerie. II. Title.
RJ47.5.C663 1991   618.92′0001′9–dc20   90-14176
ISBN 0-19-261899-7

Typeset by Downdell Limited, Oxford
Printed in Great Britain by
The Guernsey Press Co. Ltd.,
Guernsey, Channel Islands.

To all our children

Preface

Parents aim to provide a safe and happy future for their children. When, however, a child has a serious illness, their parents have to face the possible future implications, and the whole family is fundamentally affected. They have to cope with alien and traumatic situations where medical personnel, their machinery, and their medicines, seem to take centre stage. This is always difficult for parents and their children, and for the medical team trying to help them. Everyone is under stress. Death and suffering in childhood are hard for anyone to come to terms with, and practical help in handling such situations is hard to find. Indeed, health professionals often avoid facing their own emotions by hiding behind their practical roles, and parents may find some of their family and friends do the same.

This book is a collection of contributions written by parents and some teenagers, providing a very personal insight into their experience in a medical world. At the end of each chapter is a very brief explanation giving some medical background information.

The book will be helpful to all health professionals working with children and their families. There is a void in training in this field which only parents who have faced such experiences can fill. We hope the book will facilitate discussion between parents and professionals. We also hope very much that it will be of help and support to parents and children who find themselves in similar unexpected and very difficult situations. It will give them ideas of how others like them have suffered, endured, coped with, and survived the experience.

Oxford   A.C.
June 1990   V.H.

Acknowledgements

Firstly, we would like to thank all those who have supported the authors in the writing of their contributions, especially their families. We know it was not easy.

Thank you also to Dr Aidan Macfarlane whose interest and expertise has been invaluable.

A special thank you to Dr Richard Lansdown for supporting us in this venture.

Andria Fowler and Eileen Smith efficiently typed all the accounts. Many thanks to them.

Lastly, thank you to our families for keeping us going on the journey to the completion of this quest.

Contents

Contents

1

Our baby

MARIE DARBYSHIRE

My first pregnancy was a very happy time. It just 'happened'—a few comments about the possibility of expanding from a couple into a family unit at the mutual age of 26 with four years of marriage between us, and suddenly a new and uncharted world was opening up with no problem at all. Last menstrual period 25 April 1982; estimated date of delivery 30 January 1983.

Apart from a little nausea early on in the pregnancy and car sickness throughout, I was really well. I didn't even mind the nausea—it validated everything, somehow. I bloomed, I was emotionally fulfilled. I felt our baby move at 18 weeks. He was very placid, and I knew somehow that he had a pleasant nature.

I was so well that I was only under GP care, and I carried on working until I was 34 weeks pregnant. Christmas came and went. The New Year came and went. We were slowly getting the room ready and accumulating all the things that our baby would need. I prayed for a healthy baby, and said that I didn't mind which sex. Deep in my heart I wanted a little boy, but I didn't think I could possibly be so lucky. We had our own name for him. We were both teachers, and the name was one by which many classroom rogues happened to be called at that time. Not that we would dream of giving him that name in reality, of course . . .

On Monday, 10 January 1983, I decided to visit a friend who lived an hour's drive away. I took my husband to school as it was on my way. He could then share some of the driving on the way back, as I was starting to feel a bit tired, I had to admit. I blamed it on Christmas, and on the end of the pregnancy. That particular day

I'd woken up with a jump at about 5.30 a.m. as if I'd had a bad dream.

All went according to plan: I was definitely slightly under par, but delighted to see my friend. She cooked me a lovely lunch, but after having it I noticed that I had indigestion, or one of the non-specific pregnancy stomach-aches. Something wasn't quite right. I wasn't bothered though—I'd had such a relatively trouble-free time; I was determined to accept a few aches and pains as part of being heavily pregnant. It was probably waking up so early that did it. I just needed more rest.

The stomach-ache got worse towards mid-afternoon. It was a constant pain. I hoped I wasn't getting a tummy bug—there had been a few about. The baby hadn't really moved today but that was nothing unusual. Sometimes he'd sleep all day and shuffle during the night. I started to feel a bit sick, and was glad when it was time to go and fetch my husband. I smiled and waved goodbye to my friend and excused any lack of spirits on my part by saying that I was really tired. I drove for forty minutes or so and staggered into his school.

'I feel awful', I said. 'I just feel as though I want to curl up in a ball. You drive. I must go to bed. I don't really know what's happening. I didn't think that labour was supposed to start like this. The pain comes and goes a bit, but mostly it's there all the time.'

We got home at about 5.45 p.m. I crawled up to bed, wanting nothing to eat or drink. I did curl up in a ball. It hurt. It wouldn't stop hurting. 'I think something must be happening', I managed to say. 'Please phone them and say you are bringing me in.'

It was 6.30 p.m. My husband collected my bag. I crawled to the car. I couldn't stand up properly, it hurt so much. We got to the hospital at 7.15 p.m. I said I couldn't walk. The porters got me a wheelchair and wheeled me into the delivery suite. As they helped me to climb on to the bed, three things happened simultaneously: a large amount of bright red blood passed through my vagina; I vomited; and I collapsed, totally unable to lift myself out of the chair.

The examination followed. The fetal stethoscope. No heartbeat detected for the baby. The heart tracing (ECG). Same result. My husband being taken away for a few minutes. A face and voice explaining to me that my baby might have died, but it was just possible that it was still alive, and that I would be taken for a scan. I was bleeding and bleeding. Vomiting. The scan showed that my baby was dead. The pain was go great. I drifted into unconsciousness.

Another face, another voice. My husband was with me sometimes. The grief. Our grief. The crazy grief.

I'd been put under a consultant and was told I would have to deliver the baby normally, but before that I needed blood transfusions as I'd lost so much blood. I begged for a Caesarean section. To go through with delivering a baby knowing that it had died sometime within the last few hours—to give birth to death knowing all the time that I was doing it and that it was *our baby*! They said that wouldn't be possible as I'd lost too much blood, and was very ill myself. There was no choice. Part of me wanted for him never to leave my womb, his home.

The blood transfusion began. I was allergic to the first unit transfused. More panic. My priest was sent for. More units were transfused. Things calmed down. Our baby boy was born at 4.00 a.m. He was baptized. He was so, so, beautiful. He weighed 6 lb 6 oz. He had black hair. Someone took a photo. He was taken away. I was put in a room on my own to sleep, which I did for about three hours. When I woke up, I remembered: it wasn't a dream, it had happened. My husband, my comforter, had gone home. I cried from a depth which I never knew I had. I cried for a long time, as I was to cry many, many more times. I wanted my baby, my beautiful baby. If that wasn't possible then I wanted to be released from this suffering into nothingness.

I asked to see him again. So tiny, so perfectly formed, so beautiful, so perfect, so calm, peaceful, and so dead.

I was visited by the consultant who explained to me that I had had a concealed antepartum haemorrhage–placenta abruptio, and what all this meant. The placenta had just blown off—totally—a one in a million chance. Cause unknown. The baby was probably normal, but would I let them do a post-mortem just to make sure.

I said that I wouldn't, I had visions of my beautiful, perfect baby being dissected. It was explained to me that it would simply be a small, neat slit in the chest, and that he wouldn't look disfigured. In the end I agreed. I'm glad I did, really, it confirmed what I already thought I knew: he was normal.

A week in hospital. A room on my own. A few visitors. A wonderful husband who guided my thoughts briefly towards other topics from time to time. Our shared grief. No baby. Dead baby. Died in me. Did I kill him? Breasts full of milk. Repeated screams, 'I WANT MY BABY!'

Home. Letters. Cards. My mother staying. Our baby's funeral. Just his parents, three priests, and him. The tiny coffin going in the big black hole. I want to be in there with him, Oh God! Throw some daffodils on top of the coffin. Keep one and press it. I love you from the same depths that all the grief is coming from. I want you. Husband, grieving and helping.

Going out. Facing people. Hiding. Explaining. Avoiding. Being stared at. Crying so many tears. Embarrassment.

Certain things helped in the initial stages of grief—others took longer. My husband helped by being there, sharing and comforting. My faith helped, though at certain moments I've hated God for taking my baby. Some of my friends put their discomfort and embarrassment to one side, shared my emotions and took their lead from me. They made the effort to see me when I didn't want to see them. Some people were thoughtful enough to write their sympathy —you then have control as to when to open yourself up to receive their sympathy instead of it being thrust upon you verbally.

The baptism and the funeral of our baby and the priests involved helped me in my grief. He was classed as a full-term baby, and was of course baptized with the name by which we had always known him. There was also the student nurse who cried with me when he was brought back for me to see the next morning. (I wish I'd been encouraged to hold him.) I don't know her name, but she gives me some of my most powerful, comforting memories. When no one else has seen your baby except your husband, yourself, and the medical staff, you need those people to react and share in the mourning. It is a further proof of his existence which you desperately need, and it can help to diminish your sense of feeling ridiculous. It was so important for me to see him and have a photo of him, which I propped up on my bedside table (I wish I had more). It helped when friends reacted 'normally' when I showed them his photo and they said how beautiful he was.

I received a lovely letter (totally unexpected) from the mother of an acquaintance, describing her experiences of giving birth to a stillborn baby. This did begin to help me to feel less of a freak, and was all the more valuable as she was someone that I knew. I feel that this benefited me more than joining a support group would have done as, for me, the artificiality of that situation would have been difficult to cope with. It helped to be able to visit his grave whenever I wanted. Also at that early stage, my mother, who some-times seems to make heavy weather out of trivial inconveniences, displayed the most amazing amount of courage, strength, and resilience.

Other things also helped in the healing process, although it took a longer time either for them to happen or to take effect. My doctor signed me off work until I felt emotionally strong enough to go back and face everybody. My employers accepted me back at my former post in the middle of April, a few weeks after I had resigned, feeling that I'd never be able to face everyone.

It helped me to exercise to get my body back into shape. I knew that although my body was responsible for the death of my baby, I had not been at fault in any way.

We decided to move house. This encouraged us to look to the future, instead of always to the past. I was also helped by having a car, and with it the freedom to drive and think. Material possessions can be of some help through the healing process, although they're not an end in themselves.

I was able to conceive again easily, becoming pregnant three months later. Although this was accompanied by a great deal of anxiety, I had one very clear objective which perhaps bordered on an obsession—to have a baby. This was a tremendous contrast to my low-key approach to pregnancy and childbirth the first time around. The knowledge of my new pregnancy also helped to anaesthetize me to the pain of seeing my friends' newborn babies, which were starting to appear by then.

Time gradually took away the raw, bleeding pain and replaced it with another pain which is generally easier to bear. To have been informed of this at the time, however, would have been insulting and insensitive, as it would have appeared that my grief was being trivialized. Throughout, there was a sense of kindness which emanated towards me from other people, and my husband was able to be so strong.

Some things did not help.

Sometimes the reactions of medical staff sounded mechanical. I knew I was 'different', it therefore seemed important to be treated differently. A few doctors appeared *so* unemotional and distant that I thought that perhaps I was mad. I needed a brief display of sensitivity from every doctor who came into contact with me during my stay in hospital. If there was no acknowledgement of my grief, however brief, it was a denial of the existence of my baby. The more 'status' someone had (medically speaking), the more vital the need for this acknowledgement became.

Sometimes I heard babies cry in hospital. I didn't know if they were real or dreams and the grief was overpowering.

The milk in my breasts emphasized my loss.

If people stared at me when they met me for the first time afterwards, I felt desperately insecure and full of panic.

When I saw other mothers out locally with their prams who'd been at parentcraft classes with me, I remember experiencing panic and embarrassment and hiding or dodging behind parked lorries or buses to avoid them.

It was difficult when people, either in a social or work situation, tried to be kind by directly telling me how sorry they were. I might just have been managing to concentrate on something else for five minutes (a massive achievement in the early days) and it destroyed everything I'd built up and just left me with a sense of desperation and helplessness.

I felt guilt. It was my body that killed my baby. Although it was an involuntary act, that fact remains.

I felt 'different', a freak, a failure who couldn't give birth to a live baby.

When the health visitor came for a chat at home about a month afterwards, it seemed (perhaps mistakenly) so easy to put on an act of everything being under control, and I felt slightly patronized.

When I made the first hospital visit for my next pregnancy, I had to recall the story of my first pregnancy. The memories of my last time there were already powerful enough, without having to give a blow by blow account of it to a stranger who had access to the previous notes.

Some people told horror stories about the awful things that had happened to people they'd known who were pregnant. This certainly did not help, especially next time I was pregnant.

Some people who said 'I've been through exactly the same thing' actually meant they'd been through a miscarriage. I felt that a stillbirth was different from a miscarriage, and this was later confirmed by personal experience.

A further chapter opened in my life when I became pregnant again, about four months after the death of my baby. This time there was no question of GP care only—it was joint care, and I was back on the consultant's books again.

Unfortunately this pregnancy only lasted for 13 weeks. I started bleeding, and was taken to hospital, where it was explained to me that my hormone levels showed that this fetus had died in the womb, and that the contents of the womb needed to be removed (D&C). I insisted on reassurance that it was definitely dead. Then the D&C went ahead. My husband was at a tennis match and unable to be contacted. I missed him. I only spent one day in hospital. Another loss to face. We bought a new car and went on holiday to the Lake District. They both helped a bit.

I only had one period before I became pregnant yet again. The idea of contraception seemed ludicrous somehow. I was mildly chastened by my GP, but my consultant did not say anything. He explained to me in detail what had happened during my second pregnancy—how the 10-week scan had picked up the fact that the baby wasn't developing normally and the heart wasn't developing, and how they hadn't informed me, but had allowed nature to take its course. (The correct decision, as far as I was concerned.) It was wonderful to have a detailed explanation.

My third pregnancy progressed. I was constantly tired, nauseous, over-emotional and very anxious. A pregnancy did not equal a baby for us, so we got nothing ready. As the pregnancy progressed, I felt the urge to start making preparations for this baby's arrival, but my husband put his foot down, explaining that he'd had to dismantle everything and put it all away after the first time, and couldn't go through it all again.

My consultant was wonderful, a knight in shining armour. He was an excellent communicator, and to me he communicated trust in his judgement and skill, reassurance, and a sense of partnership. His listening skills were excellent, and my fears (and probably neuroses) were never ridiculed. Everything was explained to me that I could possibly want explained, and I was always treated with dignity and respect. It helped more than anything could have done. I never felt that anything was happening to me that I could not control with him—very important in view of the lack of control and powerlessness that I experienced at the end of my first two pregnancies.

I gave birth to a baby boy on 4 May 1984, four weeks early. Due to a panic on my part about a vaginal delivery, a Caesarean section was performed using an epidural anaesthetic.

My partnership with the consultant did not end here. Two and a half years later I was again pregnant. I had the same consideration and care, as I was once again riddled with anxiety, and all went well until about 30 weeks. 'Shall we aim for a vaginal delivery this time?' he said. A big lump was in my throat, my eyes were burning and tears were spilling out.

'I know you'll probably think I'm absolutely cuckoo', I said, 'but I don't think I can do it. I'll make up any stories I can to make them give me a section because I know they won't take any risks with my past history. I'll say anything, because I'm locked into thinking that anything that's delivered vaginally will be dead or quickly die. I know that it's all illogical and irrational because my first baby died before I got to hospital, but my fear and past memories are more powerful than the logic. I'm sorry.'

I was crying hard now.

He understood.

The pressure started to diminish.

We agreed that a vaginal delivery was our aim, but he was able to acknowledge my deep fears.

He communicated to me verbally and non-verbally that he understood. For the following two months he continued to explain my test results and graphs, reassuring me that all my results indicated that everything was going well. I still agreed to try for a vaginal delivery and we (possibly 'he', but he made it feel like 'we') agreed that I should be induced a week or so before the baby was due.

He wasn't there himself, but all went according to plan, and thanks to the confidence he had instilled in me, my third little boy was born vaginally with no problems on 21 April 1987.

Thank you. I never thought I could do it.

OUR BABY

Sometimes a baby is lost during pregnancy because of the presence of a lethal abnormality, but often a stillbirth is the loss of a normal child. One of the aims of antenatal care is to recognize 'danger signs' in pregnancy. Sometimes a baby may not grow well or there may be concerns over the mother's health, and an early delivery may avert a stillbirth. Usually, though, the baby's death is unheralded and sudden.

In England and Wales in the years 1985–1987 between five and six of every one thousand babies were stillborn.

V.H.

2

Jackie

HILARY BARRETT

Birth

'Not my baby—dear God, not my baby'.

I was 25 weeks pregnant, in intense pain, and terrified. A nagging discomfort all that busy Sunday had gradually become a niggling low ache. About 6.30 in the evening, I had been shocked to see blood on my underwear when I went to the loo—but it wasn't much, not worth worrying about, not nearly as much as there had been two months before.

A quick call to our GP confirmed that it was probably nothing serious, but this baby was special, conceived after five years of wanting and failing, tests, and fertility treatments, so I obeyed orders and went to bed while my husband Bob cooked our Sunday dinner. It was a lovely giggly silly meal, pork chops, peas, and boiled potatoes. Even now, after ten years, my memory replays clearly the fun of sitting up in bed trying to cut a slightly tough chop, the gravy threatening to run off the plate at every lurch of the tray.

I was uncomfortable that night, the ache gradually got worse. I tried grumpily to work out how I would fit in a doctor's appointment with my office commitments the next day. Sleep would not come, though Bob snored peacefully beside me. Something was obviously wrong, but it would only be an infection of some sort, the last thing I needed in the frantically busy three weeks before I stopped work.

At 2.30 a.m. my movements in the bed woke Bob from a heavy

sleep. I was in pain, and beginning to feel scared by its strength.

'I'm going to ring the doctor' he decided.

'No', I insisted, 'You can't call out a GP in the early hours of a Monday morning!'

An hour passed, the pain becoming worse, rising and falling. Bob rang the Medical Centre number. By chance our own doctor was taking the overnight duty, and he agreed to come out.

4 a.m.—the doctor has examined me, seen the pain rise and recede. Usually he smiles as he talks, but not now. 'Hospital', he says, and takes Bob aside. The nightmare begins, doubts harden, it's the baby, he's dying, NOT MY BABY, DEAR GOD, NOT MY BABY.

(Long afterwards, Bob told me that the doctor had warned him that the baby could not survive being born so early, the only hope was for the hospital to be able to stop my labour.)

An ambulance is coming. The hospital is forty miles away, across a county border. It seems that the doctor has had some difficulty finding an ambulance crew willing to work past the end of their shift to take me there.

The pain comes strongly now, each wave harder than the last. My body fights to protect the child in me. NOT MY BABY, DEAR GOD, NOT MY BABY.

5 a.m.—the ambulance is here. Pain hits me as I walk downstairs, and my legs dissolve. I sag on to a stair and almost fall. It is a relief to be in the ambulance, lying down again, a quiet strong voice reassuring me as the next incredible pain wells up.

Bob is to follow by car and then lead the ambulance through the side-roads to the hospital. Being out-of-area, this ambulance driver has never been there before. As the ambulance doors shut I know that this is my fight; only I can protect our baby now.

Each bump in the road triggers violent pain. I retreat into a core inside myself, desperately trying to hold the pain away from the baby. My mind screams with every lurch of the ambulance but my voice whispers 'NOT MY BABY, NO, NOT MY BABY'. The ambulanceman is with me, his hand on me, a focus of comfort and strength.

6.15 a.m.—Time slips, the pain seems to have lasted forever.

Suddenly we are in a building, moving fast, faces appear and go away, new voices in the background.

They change my clothes, put a hospital gown on me. My arms will not obey me, the room is out of focus. I cannot hear what they say to me, the words will not make sense. A corner of me is disgusted by my weakness and panic.

One clear voice intrudes through the fog, calling my name.

'Hilary! Hilary! Your baby has to be born. If you want it to live you'll have to help us'. Yes, my baby is still alive, I WANT HIM TO LIVE.

'I don't know what to do.' My voice seems to shout but they bend close, make me repeat it. Now I am really terrified. My baby is about to be born. I know nothing about it, I have not even started antenatal classes yet, and its life or death depend on me. The pain seems to increase in waves without decreasing between them. I am back in that tiny space inside myself, closing off an impossible reality.

A calm face is close to mine, smiling but with anxious eyes. Grey hair just shows under a sort of shower-cap; the face is younger than the greyness suggests. 'It's all right, just do what I tell you, your baby has a chance.' My eyes hold the cap, now moving away but still near, as the trolley moves again into a room full of hospital equipment.

Hands guide me—orders, scarcely understood—pain even sharper and longer, swelling until I scream helplessly inside myself—then nothing, suddenly it stops, blissful peace. No, they want more, 'You've got to help your baby'—force it out, hate it for the pain, feels like final rejection.

A baby tinier than a doll dangles in the air above me, limp.

The same voice, calm but commanding. 'It's a girl, look at your baby, we must take her away now.' He can't be a girl, that's our son; we've only thought about boys' names.

Exhausted, I cannot fight any more. There's a sea of faces at the end of the trolley. They're wrapping the little body in tin foil, giving it oxygen through a miniature mask that still covers most of its face.

It is taken away; alive or dead, I cannot tell.

Baby Barrett was born at 7.47 a.m. on Monday, 26 November 1979, at 25 weeks and 3 days gestation.

I am empty, numb, useless. There is no joy in this birth, only shock and disbelief. It falls to Bob to telephone our mothers and convince them that the unthinkable has happened: our baby, due next March, is born. Their worlds shatter with ours.

A nurse comes into the room, in Delivery Suite, where I wait blankly. 'Your baby's in skibboo.' What? 'Do you want to see your baby?' I'm still trying to understand 'skibboo', my stupid brain will only tell me that it rhymes with 'Timbuctoo'! The nurse sits beside me on the bed, looks a bit like my little sister. More insistent, 'Surely you want to go and see your baby?' No, yes, I WANT MY BABY, feel tears come and haven't the strength even to control them. Someone else comes in, it's 'Doctors' Rounds' now—we can't go, it will have to be later. Bob has seen our baby, he will only say that it is very small. He goes away, has to go to work. He looks awful.

Day 1

I am taken upstairs, to Level 6, mothers who have had their babies. A six-bed bay is empty, my bed is by the window. Someone has mentioned 10.30. 'Get some rest, have a sleep', they say kindly, and leave me. I sit on the side of the bed and stare unseeingly across a faraway landscape of green fields and toy houses; other people in another world going to work on their normal Monday mornings.

Babies cry all round me and I ache with emptiness, too drained even to weep, too tense for any thought of rest or sleep. It would be bliss to have someone to talk to, someone with time to listen, but the ward staff are busy with real mothers and their proper babies.

A nurse arrives eventually—with a wheelchair! Surely not for me? But yes, apparently it is necessary. I feel an absolute fool and a fraud, the first human feelings for several hours.

Lifts—corridors—then heat, hospital equipment, and babies— surely I should know which one is mine, isn't that supposed to be a maternal instinct?

This one? No feeling towards it, I'm just numbly sorry for the tiny scrap. Listen, you fool, they're talking to you. Will it live? WILL IT LIVE?

Very small, 780 grams, one pound twelve ounces they say. Everyone is being so kind, and I am so confused. Name? James Robert, no, it's a girl, we haven't thought about girls' names. I cannot accept that our son is a girl.

'If she gets through the first 24 hours . . .' It will probably die, I can hear it in your voice. No, baby, don't die, we want you, we need you.

I need to hold it in my arms, tell it how much we care, tell it how sorry I am that it is not still safely inside me. I am not numb now, I am exploding inside with the need to reach out to this baby. 'Touch her', the nurses say. I cannot—its separateness from me is like a screen round it, a barrier that it will not let me cross. My mind cries out to it, baby, we care, don't die.

The nurse must get back to the ward, so I must return, too. I hate the wheelchair, decide that it will not confine me again. Can you not understand? I want to be with this baby while it is alive. I can see its struggle, I feel death so close to it, I want to protect it.

We go back to the ward. Again I am numb, acutely aware of being physically empty. I feel like a useless spare part. How long before I can escape downstairs again? Why do I feel I have to ask permission to go, like some schoolkid needing to be excused? Why do the ward staff seem reluctant to give that permission? No, I do not need an escort. I promise not to fall over or do anything equally feeble.

Later I am moved to a single room on Level 6, a kind thought so that I will not be disturbed or upset by mothers with their babies. It increases my feeling of isolation and numbness.

We need to find a name for 'it'. I look again at our newborn baby with the old, old face and feel that it already has a name, we just have to guess what it is. If we guess wrongly, it dies. Bob wants to call it 'Christina Franchesca', a lovely lilting name, but I argue that it's too big a name for this tiny infant. Deep inside me, I acknowledge that I don't want to give a favourite name to a child who will die. Finally we choose 'Jacqueline'. Long afterwards, my twin sister reminds me that this was the name of my best doll when we were very small.

We give her my name, Hilary, for her second name. When she dies, she will take a part of me with her. Suddenly I know that she is my child, my baby, our first daughter. We go to her and tell her the names we have given her. A nurse writes them on her card. I look at her and call to her silently, over and over, 'Jackie, Jackie, Jackie'. She lies so still, her eyes sealed shut. We have only seen the left eye open a crack so far, the right one is still shut like a newborn kitten's. She looks almost plump, and strangely peaceful.

She is so tiny, so vulnerable, so alone. Her skin is covered with fine pale fur, her eyebrows are sketched by the direction of the hairs. Now that she has a name I can think of her as a baby girl, our daughter, and the confusion in my mind is less. Don't die, Jackie, please don't die.

She has lived for one hour—two hours—six hours—twelve hours. I go to sleep eventually, unable to stay awake any longer, totally empty and drained.

Day 2

I woke suddenly at 6.30 next morning. The nurse coming through the door of my room was the one from Delivery Suite, still wearing her 'shower cap'.

'I've just seen your baby, she's alive, she's survived the night.' That wonderful nurse disappeared before I could hug her for bringing the only news I needed to hear. The ward staff had not thought to ring the Special Care Baby Unit (SCBU, the 'skibboo' of yesterday—I'm learning the jargon fast), and check on my baby. Later, I told them the good news.

Again I had to wait until after 'Doctors' Rounds' before I could go to SCBU and be with Jackie.

Later that morning I was introduced to a fiendish contraption that was to rule my waking life for the next four months—the breast pump. If any new mother has any shred of dignity left after the experience of giving birth, this machine, this Iron Cow, will remove it. At the first painful attempt I achieved less than 5 ml of milk. 'Try to use it every four hours, it will stimulate your milk supply.' At one stage, when Jackie was about three months old, I was feeding not only my own baby but also six babies in a Special Care Baby Unit in another hospital! The daily tally of milk 'production' became a challenge, a focus of frustration. It was the only thing that I, and I alone, could do for my baby.

The only good thing about the communal breast pump, in the claustrophobic cupboard of a room in the SCBU area, was the social gathering as we queued to use it. For a few minutes we were Mums with a common problem, new babies in trouble, and we supported each other through the dramas and traumas of each tiny life.

Day 3

Queuing to use the breast pump the following morning, I decided to go down the observation corridor and have a quick look at Jackie. She was the furthest baby from the observation window, and I am not very tall, so I had to stretch and peer to see any part of her through the jungle of equipment round her cot and the others in between us. There was some activity round the baby nearest to the window, doctors and nurses were busy round its cot, but they were simply an inconvenience to me, partly blocking my view of Jackie.

Suddenly one of the nurses noticed me at the window, said something to the doctor, and lowered the venetian blind on the window.

It was the end of the world for me. I only wanted to see my baby, but even that had been taken away. That feeling of devastation, loss, grief has not lessened with time, it is still deeply painful to recall it. I sagged against the wall, I sobbed all the tears that had been dammed inside me since Jackie's birth.

Gradually I was aware of someone beside me. I was crouched on the floor and she was sitting uncomfortably beside me, saying something.

The doctors and nurses had been concerned that I might be upset by seeing whatever they were doing to the other baby. They had lowered the venetian blind as a kind and considerate action. This nurse had come into the observation corridor on another errand, about ten minutes later. She was surprised to see someone apparently collapsed by the wall, she did not recognize me as the 'face' at the observation window or as Jackie's mum. She spoke to me several times before she had any response, and even then it was not very coherent.

These things I know now; at the time, that was the beginning of my 'out-of-control' day. It frightened me; my lack of knowledge of the birth process included a lack of information about the after-effects of giving birth. I was not expecting 'baby-blues', the weepy day, call it what you will. By that afternoon I had wept all over Jackie, all over my lunch, and in front of at least two nurses who were genuinely too busy to stay and be drowned. An unsuspecting Staff Nurse came to ask me some routine question during the 'rest time' that afternoon, and stayed to help me. I believe that she probably saved my sanity. She told me that my reaction was normal, that it had a cause, that it would pass. She let me talk at last, and stayed to listen. Then she put me to bed like a small child, with care and concern. I woke much later as a sane, controlled adult again.

I have recorded in detail my own immediate reactions at the time of Jackie's birth. I look back on them as if they belong to a different person, yet I know they are my memories, painfully vivid even as Jackie passes her tenth birthday. I am normally considered a strong-minded, positive, controlled individual. I cope with crises; people turn to me for help; I am intelligent and capable. At the time of Jackie's birth I was thirty years old, fairly mature for first-time motherhood, with a demanding freelance job developing and running industrial training programmes.

Technology and wires

From the first minutes after her birth, Jackie was surrounded by machines, drips, wires, tubes. By the second day of her life she was under ultraviolet lights to combat jaundice, and her face was

almost hidden under enormous eye-pads. The plumpness of the
first twenty-four hours fell away, and by the third day of her life
she was a skeleton covered with dark skin. Her weight fell from 780
grams at birth to about 610 grams by day 3.

The wires and tubes never bothered us as parents, the bleeping
and clicking machines were soon familiar friends. Nurses had tact-
fully tried to prepare us for the first visual impact of SCBU, but
our anxiety at the time had mostly blocked any understanding of
what they were saying.

Bob, my husband, regarded the machines with professional
interest—his career is with computers. I saw a scene that was no
more unreal than the frozen snapshots of the past few hours, that
my numb mind was still replaying. When I finally saw my baby,
about four hours after she was born, I focused on the only part of
the scene that was at all familiar. I cannot recall what wires or tubes
were attached to her when I first saw her, but I have a vividly clear
memory of how she looked, of the smells and sounds of SCBU, of
the pale blue smock of a nurse standing very close to me and telling
me about her.

On most occasions when we walked into SCBU there was a nurse
or doctor at Jackie's bedside, willing to talk about her in as much
detail as we wanted to hear. We were always encouraged to ask
questions. No matter how mundane or technical they might be,
they were always fully answered. It helped us to feel that we knew
what was happening to her and we could trust the SCBU staff to
tell us exactly how she was, the bad times with the good.

We had to learn a large amount of medical jargon. Working in a
technical environment, nurses and doctors naturally use abbreviations and acronyms for equipment and processes. Our endless
questions must have been irritating to them, but they always
responded with patience.

Within days we could cast a glance over Jackie's monitors and
spot the differences since we had last been with her. Oxygen levels
went up and came down, a drip might be changed slightly, the
heartbeat pattern and rate would be regular or jumpy.

We also learnt quickly to see the changes in Jackie herself.
'Watch the baby, not the numbers' was the rule. Bob, being a

computers man, believed the machines; the baby was a far more unpredictable event!

We took photographs of Jackie, not just one or two a week but reel after reel of film, hundreds of photographs, especially in those early weeks. We could not wait for a film to be developed before we started the next one. We thought that we were creating our own record of our baby, that it would be the only record of a very short life. We believed that the photographs would be all we would have to remember her by.

Crisis

Jackie clung to life.

Shortly after birth she was put on a ventilator because she was 'forgetting' to breathe; her brain and lungs were just not mature enough to keep going automatically. Within days she developed a lung infection, her lungs filled with fluid and partly collapsed. The ventilator was increasing the lung secretions so it was removed when she was four days old.

She kept going, somehow, but she was getting weaker. A doctor commented later that the only factor in her favour was that she did not have a 'patent ductus' heart problem, common in premature babies; had she had that problem too, he thought she would probably not have survived.

During the next fortnight she seemed to sink. I started a notebook when she was one day old, recording each day what she did and what was done to her. My rule to myself was that it had to contain at least one positive observation each day. It was my lifeline—when everything seemed hopeless, I could look back and see that she had opened both eyes on day 6, she was 'still making progress' on day 8, I heard her cry ('like the mew of a kitten') on day 10.

She was gaunt, the still-furry skin stretched tightly over her bones. Her face often looked like a lizard's or a frog's, not like that of a human baby. Her ears were soft flaps of skin, wrinkled like cabbage leaves. Her eyes bulged even when they were shut. She could open both eyes now, but only by using the muscles of her forehead to pull up her eyelids. With her eyes shut she looked like an old, old woman. Relaxed, her face was a miniature of my grandmother's face, but my grandmother had died eight years before. She too had suffered chronic chest problems in her last three years and had been extremely thin. Watching Jackie, I often felt I was watching my grandmother.

I found myself willing her to take the next breath, timing my breathing to hers, holding my breath as she paused. The nurses told us she was 'fragile'; it meant that she would not tolerate being touched, it seemed to startle her and shock her system so that she would stop breathing and her heart would threaten to stop, too. Physiotherapy was essential to keep removing the secretions from her lungs, but it was obviously very distressing for her. She could not keep breathing afterwards, her heart-rate was very slow. I felt responsible for her suffering, guilty at wanting her to live, tormented by trying to face her death.

It was her twentieth day. We spent the afternoon watching her fight, aware of her exhaustion. Awake, she 'remembered' to breathe. The slightest sharp sound or touch on her body triggered her 'panic' reflex, she jerked, her arms and legs crabbed, she stopped breathing and her heart-rate sank. She looked bruised, as if she had been physically beaten, especially around her face. Every fifteen to twenty minutes she fell asleep and stopped breathing. The alarm on her apnoea mattress bleeped and a nurse would come and 're-start' her, flicking her foot, waking her enough to make her breathe again. Sometimes it was not enough, and it was necessary to pump air into the tiny lungs and inflate the still chest. The face-mask was no bigger than the bowl of a small teaspoon.

Late that afternoon a doctor came to talk to us. His name has faded from memory but I will never forget his face. He explained that he might have to put Jackie back on the ventilator. He described his dilemma; without the ventilator she was too tired to breathe on her own, but the tube in her lungs would increase the secretions, which could kill her. He told us that she might not live through the night.

We turned back to our desperately ill baby. That doctor had

confirmed the evidence of our own eyes; she was getting weaker as we watched her. Suddenly all the fighting of the last few days seemed so futile. I felt deeply guilty for her pain and her suffering. She had fought so hard, and I had done so little for her. It was unreasonable to ask more of her—but I needed her so much, it was so hard to let her go.

I prayed then, more honestly than I had ever prayed before. 'Dear God, if Jackie is going to die, please take her tonight so that she doesn't have to suffer any more. She has suffered enough, God. But if she is going to have a useful life, please God give her strength to fight this, only please don't make her linger and suffer and then die.'

I was not at that time a regular church-goer, nor was I used to praying. It just seemed to be right.

We said goodbye to our baby—not a quick temporary goodnight kiss but a farewell, in the clear belief that we would not see her alive again. She was needing almost constant attention from nurses and doctors; there was mercifully little opportunity to linger. We held her tiny hands for the last time and went home. 'There is no point in you staying,' the doctor had said, 'we will ring you . . .'

How long does such a memory remain acutely painful? I write it now through the distortion of tears, an echo of the tears I shed through that long night. The telephone did not ring. I made myself wait until 7.30 the next morning, an hour earlier than usual for my morning call to the Unit. She was on the ventilator and sleeping. She was alive.

The next three months

Days passed. 'Two steps forward and one step back' continued to be the pattern, but somehow Jackie seemed to have turned a corner. We smiled at ourselves for getting excited about her feeds of my milk increasing from 1 ml per hour to 2 ml per hour, then gradually to the huge amount of 6 ml per hour, just over a teaspoonful!

It was almost Christmas, though neither Bob nor I could raise any enthusiasm for it. He was commuting to a freelance job on the other side of London. Before Jackie's birth he had stayed in digs during the week and been home at weekends. Now he commuted daily, two hours each way on the Underground, then two or three evenings a week he drove the eighty miles to the hospital and back. On the days when he could not visit, I went in by myself or with friends. Bob was exhausted and it was affecting his work. I felt 'alive' only when I was with Jackie, time spent at home was blank.

On Christmas Day we visited Jackie in the afternoon. She was just one month old and had regained her birth-weight a few days before. She was still on the ventilator but more alert, trying to turn her head to follow movements.

Nurses in party hats greeted us as we walked into SCBU. By now we knew most of their names; all the nursing staff are known by their first names, which makes it easier to form friendships with them. Sally was wearing a doctor's dark blue overalls, several sizes too big for her, and John, the on-duty doctor (looking as if he had not slept for at least twenty-four hours) was wearing a nurse's pale blue smock. We were delighted to see that several of our 'favourite' nurses were on duty. Laura was standing by Jackie. 'Come and see, she's got her best dress on for you!' she called. There was Jackie, looking just like a 'proper' baby, wearing a tiny blue smock for the first time. There was a Christmas card to us from Jackie. I still have it, in her photograph album. Father Christmas had brought her a little rabbit, and that too is still around, rather worn and well-loved now.

Laura was doing something to Jackie so we stood back while she finished, not wanting to get in her way. 'Sit down, then', she said. I must have been slow to respond. Laura turned, her face beaming. 'Don't you want to hold your baby, then?' I sat—my legs would not stand! Suddenly Jackie was in my arms for the first time, still on the ventilator, but held against me, so tiny that she felt as if she would slip between my arm and my body, so light and fragile that it was like holding a bird. I was so huge and clumsy, so scared and happy at the same time. She was my very own baby, held in my arms, and for a few moments there was no one else in the world but us. It was the best Christmas present I have ever had. Bob held her too. Our photo of him holding her is not his favourite, he says he has a 'soppy expression' on his face. There are times when the strongest men cry.

In Jackie's room now, a tiny trinket dangles from her lampshade. Measuring only about an inch in any dimension, it is an 'angel' sitting in half a walnut shell. My twin sister Shelagh sent it to her, and us, as a Christmas present. Shelagh was living in America then and had to send it several weeks before Christmas, to arrive in time. She addressed it to the Special Care Baby Unit, with a note asking them to give it to Jackie on Christmas Day if she lived, or to hold it and not even mention it to us if she died. It has watched over Jackie since that first Christmas Day, a symbol for me of her fight to live.

Jackie improved from then. I commented to a nurse that the fairies had taken my sick baby and left another in its place—the change was so dramatic. In a strange way I believed my own joke— I was trying to adjust to a different baby. Later, I believe I even 'mourned' that first phase of Jackie's life, almost as if she had actually died and another baby had replaced her.

Four days later, on the weekend after Christmas, we made the decision to go out and order Jackie's cot and start to get her room ready at home. She was making such a fight, we had to believe at last that one day she would come home, would sleep in her cot. It was our act of faith in her. We tried to explain to the shop assistant that we did not know even which month we might need the cot, it could be any time from about March. The assistant was so dubious that she called her supervisor. The picture of Jackie (always in my handbag) came out. We told her Jackie's story. It was the beginning of a pattern which has threaded through Jackie's childhood, partly a recognition that Jackie has always been 'different' from other children, partly a need in me to talk about her and 'excuse' her difference—I am aware that I tell her story as a premature baby far less often now that she is not noticeably different from other children of the same age.

Jackie was taken off the ventilator, promoted back to an incubator, and promoted into the 'less intensive' room as being the least ill baby in the 'hot' room! Each step forward was a triumph, but at the same time a cause for concern—would she keep breathing on her own, would she get the same care in the next room, was she really ready for 'promotion'? If those young nurses had known how critically I watched their handling of my baby, they would have dropped her in fright! I hated the incubator. It was a physical barrier between Jackie and me. Logically it was better for her, and I could see that she was improving and did not need such intensive nursing. But the mother in me wanted her as close as possible, and the incubator kept me at a distance.

The visits were magical when, for a few short minutes, we could take Jackie out of her incubator and cuddle her. In my notebook the first few occasions are recorded in capital letters. I could pretend that she was my own baby, I could shut my mind to the oxygen line and the wires and her miniature fragile body and I could hold my real living child in my arms.

She was 54 days old. We were greeted with great excitement as we went into the unit that day. 'The doctors gave Jackie three cheers this morning', my notebook records. She had passed the one kilogram milestone at last; she actually weighed as much as a bag of sugar! Eight doctors had stood round her incubator clapping and cheering, making so much noise that all the nurses in the Unit had looked up to see what the fuss was about.

Now she behaved more and more like a real baby and it was harder and harder to leave her. One evening I finally could not bear it. She was bright and happy, a lovely baby. Bob needed to get home to sleep but I desperately needed my baby. Visiting time sped by. The clock was my greatest enemy. 'Time to go', he said, for the sixth or seventh time. Tears came (how many tears were shed in those months). It was impossible, I could not leave her, I had my arms round the incubator as she lay innocently inside gazing up at me. I cried, sobbed, completely lost control. Nurses came, I think— it is a blurred memory, only the feel of the hard incubator and the picture of her tiny face are focused, with the intense pain of my need to be with her. We went home—but it hurt.

At that time, when Jackie was in SCBU and we were at home, it felt as if she and I were joined by a length of elastic. When we were apart it stretched to its fullest extent, constantly pulling me back towards her. I always drove too fast along the motorway to the hospital on the days when I made the journey alone. Going home was purgatory and many times I had to pull over on the hard shoulder, unable to see through my tears. Why I never crashed the car I will never know, it must have been by the grace and skilled driving of other motorists.

In spite of the anxieties, my breast milk continued. The Iron Cow was now a natural part of my daily routine, at home or at the hospital. The wonderful day came when Jackie first attempted to suck from a bottle. She was 66 days old, and by then 35 weeks gestation. To my terror, I had the task of feeding her with her first bottle—we were beginners together! Perhaps every first-time Mum feels this way about the first bottle-feed. Does everyone record the momentous occasion with a photograph too?

She only managed about 10 ml from the bottle, then she was exhausted. Later, a nurse described a tiny baby's effort to drink milk from a bottle as 'like an adult trying to run up six flights of stairs'. Watching Jackie's reactions, we knew what she meant.

Now Jackie was a little character. One morning when I rang SCBU as usual at 8.30 a.m., the nurse on duty told me she was 'roaming round her incubator, starving hungry, looking for her breakfast'.

She sucked on everything and anything. She gazed around her, fixed her eyes on objects or faces and stared at them. She still needed extra oxygen, but as she approached ten weeks old the amount had been gradually reduced to 23 per cent. Being now very active but still very tiny, around 1300 grams, she managed to 'escape' from headboxes regularly. It had become a joke in the Unit and we were very relaxed about it, though she quickly became very pale and weary without her oxygen.

She had another bottle-feed, then another, usually given by Bob or me. She was 74 days old, a lovely active 'real' baby, beginning to look quite plump, able to be dressed in little smocks. I changed her nappy and started to bottle-feed her. Suddenly she began to choke. No problem—I patted her back. She turned scarlet, then purple. Face down over my knee—never mind if she's sick—there's a nurse in the next cubicle, get help quickly. The nurse heard my shout and came running—held Jackie upside down as she turned blue—

suddenly our tiny cubicle was full of nurses and doctors. I was in a corner trying to keep out of the way, and understand what was happening at the same time.

After about a minute (or was it several hours?) Jackie was in her incubator, her smock and nappy stripped off, naked and so terribly vulnerable. She was putty grey and was not breathing on her own, hands were holding the 'penlon' mask to her face, squeezing it, flicking her hands and feet; murmuring voices were urging her to 'come on, come on'. She breathed. So did I. Slowly her skin flushed pink again. It was a nightmare reminder of the days before Christmas, and of her still-tenuous hold on life.

It had to be that day when I had travelled to the hospital with a friend who had to return by a fixed time. I could not stay with Jackie. Again I had to tear myself away from her, leave her when I most needed to be with her. Limp and pale, she lay in her incubator, a sick baby again.

I was the pale and weary one next morning. When I rang the Unit for our early report, she was apparently pink and alert, looking for her grub!

By the middle of February, 11 weeks old and about 37 weeks 'gestation', Jackie had discovered how to get attention by setting her alarms off. It's simple really, you just get your arms up inside your headbox and lift its perspex cover. Then the oxygen level alarm bleeps and a nurse comes to investigate. Jackie disliked her headbox and became increasingly restless, fighting it with her tiny fists. Eventually the great day came, she was moved into a cot with a 'lid'. The barriers between us were coming down, my baby was coming closer to me. Why then, in the photos at this time, do I suddenly look so much more strained and pale?

Her progress galloped forward. She had yet another blood transfusion, then three days later the oxygen feed was removed for the last time. Jackie was breathing only air, and was coping! I held her against me, with only her feeding tube dangling, and just cuddled her.

The next day she and I shared a fantastic experience known as 'breast-feeding'. How do you describe that first moment when your baby sucks milk directly from you? Neither of us knew what we were supposed to do, but it seemed to work.

One day later came Jackie's first bath. I expected a lesson in baby-bathing, but no, it was a demonstration of where to find a bath and how to test the water. 'There's only one basic rule', cheerful Pam explained. 'If her head goes under, do lift it out'. I must have shown my horror in my face, because she added 'they survive most things!' Here was this precious scrap, whose life they had repeatedly saved, whose progress they had agonized over with us. Now they were about to entrust her to her clumsy amateur mother, who could just as easily drown her! We survived. Jackie was not very impressed with baths. I had the distinct feeling that I was dreaming.

She was almost, but not quite, ready to come home. In hospital I felt constrained but safe. I hated leaving her but could not face the thought of the lack of expert help, constant attention, friendly monitors, in the big world outside. The day that she was due to be born dawned and passed.

A note in my book at that time sounds despairing. 'Will she ever feed properly? How many other 25½-week babies have successfully breast-fed? Is she behaving "normally"? One day, hopefully, we'll look back on this as just another "stage"—and she's only had seven attempts so far. I have plenty of milk—but is it coming down properly for her? Am I too used to the machine? She seems to suck very well, then has only taken 20 ml. "Suck" is not very strong yet. Will she ever seem "normal"?'

It was only the next day that the magic invitation was issued— 'come in for a couple of days, then take her home'. Delight— excitement—fear—panic, all at once.

She was 16 weeks old, 41 weeks 'gestation'. It felt so strange to handle her without wearing a gown. The air itself seemed dirty, her clothes were hugely too big (she still weighed only 2215 grams, 4 lb 14 oz). I felt an enormous responsibility for her, as if I had to provide the same level of care and attention that she had enjoyed in SCBU, but by myself. Her cry was a tiny mew and could not be heard from my room to the corridor, so if she cried there was only me to come to her aid. She slept well that first night, but I woke for every grunt and squirm—and she was a very noisy sleeper!

We took her home on 15 March 1980. She was in her own carry cot, in her new crib, wrapped in her own shawls and blankets. It was exactly nine days after the date she was due to be born. The next day was Mothering Sunday and it was the most perfect Mothers' Day. She really felt like 'our' baby, our first daughter, our Jackie. After one hundred and eleven days of sharing her, she was totally ours at last.

Early days

She had been home about ten days when she became unwell. Her colour was poor, she would not wake properly, she was not interested in food, she did not even wet her nappy. Frightened, I called our doctor. Nothing was obviously wrong, but he suggested taking her back to the hospital if she was not better next day. I looked at her, and thought about the long night watching her lying ill. We took her back to the hospital that same afternoon. She lay limp and listless in my arms as we walked into the Maternity reception area. She started to wriggle as we went through the swing doors into the Special Care area. She gazed round her with the first interest she had shown all day, as we sat in the parents' room waiting for a doctor to see her. Stripped naked for weighing she wee'd on the scales, then started making unmistakable signs of hunger. By the time the doctor arrived she was comfortably settled into her first good feed of the day, calm and normal. Could she possibly have been homesick for SCBU?

Onwards and upwards

I laugh at myself, as I look back at incidents during Jackie's first year. A highlight was the routine 6-months-old check at the Health Visitors' clinic. We had agreed that the six-months check was a formality for Jackie as she really could not be fitted into the conventional 'average' ratings. The verdict was that she was about two months behind their physical milestones—and I was delighted! I remember clearly the confusion of the other mums there, with their huge 'normal' 6-month-old babies. My solemn little dolly with the old-lady expression weighed only about 8½ pounds then, but was obviously neither as young as her size suggested nor as advanced as her age claimed. And I was tremendously excited because my baby was 'only' two months behind her actual-age milestones!

It was quickly obvious that Jackie's brain was much more developed than her body. Mentally she was months ahead of her physical ability, and this difference persisted. It frustrated her; even as a small baby her determination could boil over into anger when she failed to achieve something. She is still troubled by angers and frustrations that seethe inside her and erupt from time to time.

Much of the time, Jackie was fun. She was happy when she was close to me, and that suited me. She wanted to be held so that she could see what was happening, so I used to walk around with her perched on my arm or my shoulder like a parrot. Being small and light, she was easy to carry.

It caused problems at sleep time. 'Put your baby to bed and leave it to cry', the books recommend. Jackie had not read the books. If I just put her in her crib, she screamed; she howled until she was sick with exhaustion and hiccoughs, until she could hardly catch her breath; but she did not go to sleep. I could rock her to sleep in my arms eventually, when she was weary, but she would not or could not fall asleep alone. Night after night I rocked and danced her across the landing and back again, trying to get her to sleep before our bedtime. She would doze while I moved, but wake the instant I put her down. Even now she knows all the old lullabies, nursery rhymes, Girl Guide songs, popular ballads, and folk songs that I occasionally drag from the depths of my memory. Yes, she remembers them. She heard them every night when she was tiny!

We frequently went back to the hospital for follow-up checks and research tests. I looked forward especially to the research tests. It was an opportunity to talk socially, quietly, over a long time, to a doctor who knew the quirks of premature babies and would not raise eyebrows or mentally label me as a 'fussy mother' as I asked whether this or that was 'normal' for my not-normal baby. I was also able to share Jackie's progress with nurses on the Special Care Baby Unit who had cared so much about her, and this was important to me; they accepted her as a member of SCBU making tremendous progress in the big wide world outside, not as a rather odd little soul who was different from every other 'normal' baby.

She was, physically, an odd little soul. Her head was large for her body and rather flat at the sides, elongated front-to-back. Her legs and arms were short compared with her body size. She tended to sit or stand with her arms bent, elbows pulled in to her sides, hands drawn back towards her shoulders. I thought of it as her 'little-bird' pose, but when I saw a child with cerebral palsy in the same pose, it gave me cause for private concern. I never had the courage to mention that concern to a doctor. Looking back, I think I was afraid that it might be taken seriously.

For a long time she could not crawl—she 'swam' along the floor. Eventually when she did manage to find her knees, she dragged one leg, and it seemed weaker than the other when she began to walk. Her feet were rotated outwards at a 'quarter to three' position, and they could even point slightly backwards without Jackie apparently noticing. I watched, coached, encouraged, worried to myself. It is hopeless to tell a mother 'don't worry about it'. Part of caring is the concern which makes us worry. The more we care, the more we have to worry. Jackie at age 10 still walks and runs with her feet pointing outwards, giving her a clumsy gait which is not made for speed. She detests Sports Day, which highlights her lack of physical ability still.

Jackie's muscles were obviously weak and her co-ordination was slow to develop. She was a tiny child, only about 12 lb at a year old, but powerfully determined. We started to take her swimming when she was 15 months old, as an exercise to improve her co-ordination and help her breathing. By the time she was 3 she was swimming underwater, but could not manage to get to the surface. She seemed to have an unusual ability to hold her breath, for such a small child. My own explanation was that she had concentrated so much on simply taking the next breath, as a newborn baby, that she actually had more control than normal over her breathing process. Now aged 10, she holds a badge for swimming 2000 metres—eighty lengths of a standard pool.

People meeting Jackie now see a normal child. She is bright and intelligent, with a quick and quirky sense of humour. Reserved in

manner, she often seems older than her years. She is fiercely determined, a fact which proves both an asset and a liability in different
circumstances. She is musical and enjoys playing her recorder and
listening to music.

Jackie used to be very small for her age, fragile-looking, with a
'different' face shape. She changed dramatically at about 8 years
old. Suddenly she put on weight, so that now she looks quite solid,
though she is still short for her age. She wears very strong glasses to
correct long sight, but others of her age group are now having to
wear glasses, too. She is treated as a 'normal' intelligent child with
some exceptional talents and one or two inexplicable gaps.

Am I wrong, then, still to see her as an exceptional, different,
'special' child functioning beautifully within normal limits?

Thoughts and reflections

The experience of giving birth to a very premature baby and the
subsequent stresses of the four months that she spent in hospital,
changed both Bob and me. We both realized how precious and
fragile life is, we both learnt not to waste any day. Bob reacted to
the experience by needing to plan ahead and know what each day
would hold. He tries to fill each day by planning it meticulously.
The greater his stress, the more structured his future must be. I
reacted by living each day separately, trying to spend my time with
the people who mean the most to me, my baby, my family and my
closest friends. I find it difficult to get excited about planning for
next month or next year, today seems too important.

When Jackie was 5 years old and our second daughter was
newborn, Bob suffered severe depression which required a year of
medical treatment. Talking to other parents of babies who were
premature or severely ill at birth, several have experienced this
same pattern of reaction. The mother reacts immediately; emotionally she is part of the baby's fight for life, she feels responsible for
its early or troubled birth. She must come to terms quickly with her
feelings of guilt and fear, or be permanently harmed by them. The

father, however, probably goes out to work. He leaves the home
traumas and goes into his 'normal' office environment. He suffers
a strong reaction when the child is obviously 'better', or when
another similar but successful event (like the trouble-free birth of a
subsequent child) triggers the emotion that he has submerged rather
than accepted.

We are blessed with two beautiful and intelligent daughters and
we love them both dearly. Given the chance, would we have
another child? Each is a gift from God, we can only answer: Yes,
we would accept the gift and do our best to deserve it. Whatever the
problems we are given, we are also given the strength and ability to
overcome them.

JACKIE

Progress in obstetric and neonatal care has contributed to improved survival rates of premature babies. An infant who weighs more than 1500 grams at birth is now likely to survive without significant handicap. In recent years the survival of even smaller babies, born between ten and seventeen weeks before their expected delivery date, has also improved dramatically. A singleton liveborn baby without a lethal congenital abnormality weighing less than one kilogram, who is nursed on a neonatal Intensive Care Unit, now has a greater than 70 per cent chance of survival.

These extremely premature babies are, however, fundamentally different from full term and larger preterm infants. All of their organ systems—their lungs, the central nervous system, the gut, the skin, and all the regulatory pathways—are immature in structure and function. Most of these babies need intensive support from highly trained nursing and medical staff with complex equipment, so that the usual intimate contact between newborn infants and their parents is impossible to maintain. Vulnerable very low birthweight babies find handling stressful. Very premature infants may stay in hospital for many weeks, often finally being discharged around the time of expected delivery.

V.H.

3

Natalia

KRYSTYNA SWIRYDCZUK

You will never forget the words. For as long as you live, through the sad times and the happy times, those words will always come back to you. Those first words the doctor spoke to you, telling you that there was a problem with your child. The way you accept and the way you begin to deal with the situation starts with those first words you hear.

My husband and I were in our early thirties, both career-orientated professionals, expecting our second child. Our first child, a girl, was 15 months old when we started to plan our second child. We wanted two children, about two years apart, ideally a girl and a boy, but two girls would be just fine. Although our first child was born in an emergency Caesarean section, we merely accepted our healthy baby as what we had always expected. When we found I was pregnant with our second child I was 32 years old. I briefly thought of having amniocentesis, but after vaguely mentioning it to my best friend, a doctor, she told me not to worry as I was too young to really consider it, and the chances of a miscarriage were greater than those of me having conceived a Trisomy 21 baby. I let the subject drop, but when I saw my obstetrician I once again broached the subject—to get the same reply. I decided to forget about it—surely both can't be wrong?

Natalia was born vaginally and appeared to be a normal beautiful baby. I was ecstatic that I had not had another Caesarean section, and now that we had two children our family was complete. Steve was still trying to convince me that we should have three children, but we both decided to take a wait-and-see attitude. As I looked at Natalia I tried to find some family resemblances. Our first daughter had her father's chin, but I couldn't see anything definite in Natalia to say she looked like either of us. I commented on this to a close friend as she visited me several hours after Natalia's birth, but then put it out of my mind.

The following morning the paediatrician and obstetrician were late coming to see me; in fact, Steve arrived just before they came in. And within seconds I heard the words 'we suspect your child has Down's syndrome'. Mine? This can't happen to me. This must be some dreadful mistake. No this is real. God, what do I do ???? The doctor was still talking, technically, about the way they recognize the syndrome; the characteristics Natalia had; the blood work that needed to be done; the fact that Natalia did not have an intestinal blockage; that now we must watch carefully to see if she develops a heart problem; that 44 per cent of Down's babies are born with heart problems . . . 'Are you sure?' . . . 'Almost certainly'. And as I floated back into reality, harsh as it was, I heard the words 'if you are to have a handicapped child this is the best handicap to have'. How senseless those words seemed at that time.

Soon I was asking questions. What kind of heart problems might we be talking about? What do we do now? How do we take care of the child? And I was told to treat her normally, that she would be just like any other baby, perhaps easier, but we would have to be more aware.

That night alone in my hospital room I could not begin to sleep. While Steve was with me it seemed that we had the strength to handle the news, we had each other to lean on and each other to remind us that there was a lot more to our lives than our second daughter. We had our lives and our relationship, and we also had a beautiful healthy daughter we could not forget. But alone at night in my hospital bed no one could reassure me. I kept flashing back to the only Down's person I could remember—a young man, who always used to go shopping with his mother, who obviously took care of him. And I was afraid. Was that my destiny? Would I get old trying to give my child the care that no one else would give her? What would happen when I died? Or when I was in need of care myself? Panic spread over me. Depression followed. Had my life, as I knew it, come to an end?

I don't really remember what Steve said through this time. I know he was strong, I know he was positive, and I know I relied upon him to make any rational decisions that had to be made. I know I talked of adoption as an alternative, but Steve just brushed it off as part of that silly talk new mothers go through after having a baby. Post-partum depression some call it. Steve just calls it 'the hormones'. I don't remember any of the conversations, or any of the words, but I do remember the strong positive attitude of 'this is our child and we will love her just like the other'.

I do remember, very vividly, a conversation with my obstetrician the day after we were told of Natalia's Trisomy 21. After two pregnancies and deliveries with him I felt we had reached a mutual respect and understanding for one another. I blocked out of my mind that he was one of the people who had advised me against amniocentesis. I needed all the allies I could get for strength in the present situation. Steve had long taught me never to look back and never to lay blame. I was talking, rambling, about having to give up work to raise my children now. And there was silence as he looked at me and then said 'You're going back to work. Your life is not going to be any different because of this child'. I often recall these words and gain much strength from them.

The first week was hard. Waiting for the blood work to confirm our worst fears. Still hoping there was a chance that these doctors were all wrong. Trying to explain away those syndrome characteristics by recalling some relative who had a flat face, almond-shaped eyes, low set ears . . . Trying to look happy at the birth of our child as friends visited, wanting to say something but not daring to—in case saying it out loud might turn it into reality. But then the phone call came. Confirmation of Trisomy 21. Now what? Don't look back, look forward. What needs to be done? Family and friends need to be told. We need to read and learn what all this is, what is in store for us. We need to contact the local mental health authorities and get started. Where do we begin? Tears. Panic. Depression.

Slowly the news gets out, and then spreads like wild-fire. We find some people don't know what to say, and don't come close. We find many don't know what to say but come and visit, and we cry together/laugh together. Contact is made. And a few are able to say some beautiful things that stay in our hearts for ever.

And the doctors are still there. The paediatrician monitoring for heart problems, giving helpful hints in preparation for the next stage. Though breast-feeding, I should occasionally give Natalia a bottle so that she gets used to one, and when I need to wean her to go back to work, it will be a little easier. Start a little earlier with the spoon and cereal, just so it won't feel strange to her when it's time for solids. And the obstetrician, more concerned with my mental health than with my physical health, concerned about when I would be ready to return to work.

Slowly, very slowly it seemed, I turned pain and confusion into acceptance and strength. I went back to swimming when Natalia was 8 days old, and I remember swimming hard and fast, with tears in my eyes, saying 'why me? why me?' and the harder and faster I swam the less I thought about Natalia and the more I thought about me, the me I used to know. I decided we would have another child, after all, Steve always wanted three children. I challenged myself: previously I had thought two children and a career was my limit, now I stated out loud that I could handle three children, including a handicapped child, and my career. I knew that this intense desire for another child was a natural reaction to the let down of having given birth to a not perfect child, and I knew that I would reconsider that decision later.

But it wasn't all positive thinking. Far from it. Just as vividly I remember the negative thoughts. The thought of having a fatal car crash on yet another visit to the paediatrician. Wishing for it, hoping for it. The thought of a terrible incurable heart problem that would take away the responsibilities of decision-making or future caring for our child. I never knew if it was good news or not to be told that Natalia was not showing any signs of heart problems.

As other parents of Down's children called us and reached out a helping hand, all I could do was cry, sob, and their words were to no avail. I don't remember any of them now; I only remember my tears.

Upon the paediatrician's advice we immediately contacted the social workers to enrol Natalia in early childhood intervention, or infant stimulation as they called it. As we filled out all the necessary paperwork I kept holding back the tears, thinking how crazy it was that Natalia was only three weeks old and we were sending her to school. I made a big mistake in deciding I wanted to tour their facilities, and while Natalia was still new in our lives, and still an enigma. I now know it was too-too-soon to make myself walk into any kind of facility that either taught or housed handicapped persons. All I could see through my teary eyes were shortcomings and inabilities. I could not focus on the happy smiling faces who wanted to show me their lives. I apologize to them for putting them through my visit.

I went back to work and left Natalia and her sister in the capable hands of our daily babysitter. She was the lady who had taught me how to love my first daughter, how to coo, and smile, and be delighted with every action the child made. Now she showed me there was no difference between my two children as she took care of them. Through watching her I again learned how to love. Twice a week the social worker would come to our home and teach us what to do to help Natalia develop her potential to its fullest. Here was a woman who had her own small children but worked with mine because she wanted to. She loved my child and focused on the achievements. It is through these people that I, too, learnt to love my child and focus on the positive aspects of her personality and her achievements.

We received a lot of letters from family and friends after we wrote and told them of Natalia's birth, or as they found out through mutual friends. All were supportive (why write if you can't write something positive?). All made me cry while I was reading them. Some touched me more than others. My reactions to one letter were a little surprising. My best friend, the doctor who had first advised me against amniocentesis, wrote to me upon receiving word from me. I cried my way through the letter, just like all the others, but then when I put it down I remember saying 'she sounds like a doctor, not like my best friend'.

Now, almost three years later, I have gone back to that letter for the first time, to try to analyse it, and my reactions to it. It sounds less like coming from a doctor than I remember it sounding, so why did I have that reaction? Because she began to compare my child, my special child, to other Down's children she has worked with, giving me the benefit of her knowledge of the Down's population. Why did that bother me? Perhaps because I knew, that if my child was a normal child no one would tell me of the child's potential, or the problems, or the hardships that may be involved with raising that child. The paediatrician doesn't come in and say to you that you have a perfectly normal child, who, given the general population as a control, may end up with a university degree, or may drop out of school and become a juvenile delinquent, or a drug addict. Each child is an individual and we only find out his/her potential as they develop. It is normal that parents hope for their children to reach their full potential, whatever that may be. Yet here was my friend telling me about the Down's population, and what range was to be expected from a child with Down's syndrome. But all I really cared about was my child, my child as an individual. My friend was not treating Natalia as my child, an individual, but rather as a statistic. Of course my child had a limited potential, but, nevertheless there was a potential.

When I analyse my paediatrician's approach I realize that there was a heavy emphasis on my child as an individual, and second to that, emphasis on the fact that that individual had Down's syndrome and would hence have a limited potential. In retrospect, probably the most important thing that my paediatrician did in those important early days was to place such heavy emphasis on Natalia as a child first and foremost, rather than focusing on the fact that my child belonged to a population of people who were born with an extra chromosome. She made me feel like my child was an individual, worth the love and respect that any individual deserves. She made me believe that that individual would in turn love and respect me and would enrich my life in her own way. That we would live our lives in harmony rather than in conflict: without false expectations and without false hopes.

I believe very early on in my relationship with Natalia I established a mutual respect and a bond that derived from the fact that we were both individuals and would both strive to come to our full potential; not at the expense of one another, rather with the full support of one another. And it is through this mutual respect that I have grown to love and admire my child for what she is and not what she could have been.

Recently I was faced with a close friend finding out that her 6-week-old baby had microcephaly and would, as a result, have some degree of mental retardation. My reaction was of interest to me because it came so close to my being asked to write this contribution. It helped me to understand a little better where I stood in dealing with my own situation, and I found the sharing of thoughts with my friend enlightening in terms of seeing the similarities and differences of our feelings. The biggest differences between her reactions and my reactions of almost three years ago revolved around: (1) the fact that her baby was 6 weeks old when she found out there was a problem, and (2) the fact that the diagnosis left her with far less of an idea of what to expect in the future.

The difference between a mother who became bonded to her child over six weeks, versus a new mother being told of a significant problem in their child's health can be the difference between acceptance and rejection of that child. The fact that your child has a problem that other children have, and that there are support groups for both emotional and informational help for your specific illness or problem is comforting. When the parents leave the doctor's office most of their questions will be answered by these fellow parents and most of their fears alleviated by them.

Natalia is almost 3 now. We have another child in our family, a baby boy who just turned 1. We went on to have another child to 'round-out' our family. We felt that both Natalia and our older daughter would benefit from another sibling in the family. In my own mind I know that I have greatly benefited from having another child. After Natalia was born, whenever a friend had a healthy baby, instead of being happy for them I was jealous and bitter. I did not have positive memories associated with childbirth or Natalia's early days as a baby. They were always clouded by the fact that she had Down's syndrome. Now I remember the joys of newborn babies again, and the miracle of birth.

At work I am considered confident and self-assured. That confidence and self-assurance comes from my being a mother, and in particular being Natalia's mother. Natalia is keeping her half of the bargain I made with her—that she would let me remain an individual and would help me to develop to my fullest. I hope I can keep my end of the bargain with her.

I now look at our dealings with the medical profession. We have moved and left the town where those doctors practise. But neither my husband nor I will ever forget them. For everyday family practice I have chosen a paediatrician who comes recommended by parents with Down's children: a man who treats the children equally, and one who knows the special tests and warning signs to look for in the Down's population. For any specific needs he refers me to a specialist, who always makes me feel that he sees far worse things in life than the problems I bring him. But he still has the time to sit down and discuss my problem in detail with me. I always leave feeling educated and relieved. I feel the key is always to have the situation explained as best as we, the laypersons, can understand it. So that we feel we are part of this caring team, and always to keep the diagnosis in perspective.

I look at our dealings with the social worker, the speech therapists, the occupational therapists. Each of them treats Natalia as an individual and praises her achievements. We don't discuss her as part of the Down's population, we discuss her as an individual with specific needs. We try not to label her or categorize her, although sometimes the system forces us into it, when we have to fill out the mountains of forms. We are always careful to focus back in on her as an individual.

I go back through my husband's journal, written at the time of Natalia's birth, and find a few surprises. He thought I was fairly strong through it all. I don't remember myself like that. The first week or two he wrote: 'Natalia really seems normal, you know, like a baby . . . but I guess she won't be for long'. I want to laugh. If there is one thing we now know, looking back, it is that every day she becomes more normal and closer to our expectations of her. Our expectations have changed, but she has also always exceeded our expectations. I will never forget the words and the look on

Steve's face on Natalia's first birthday: 'I never thought you would be this much fun, Natalia'. And these feelings have increased. That doesn't mean that I am not afraid of the future. I am always afraid of the unknown. But I also know that by the time the future comes we will be ready for it.

NATALIA

Human cells usually contain 46 chromosomes, separate strands of genetic material. These are made up of 23 pairs—one of each pair from the mother and one from the father. One in 600 live-born babies has an extra chromosome 21. These babies have in common some of a well-known group of physical features and medical and developmental difficulties known as Trisomy 21 or Down's syndrome. For an individual mother the chances of giving birth to a baby with Trisomy 21 increases with her age. The risks are a little over one in 2000 for a mother in her twenties, but greater than one in a 100 for a mother in her forties. None the less, most parents of infants with Trisomy 21 are in their twenties, since more women have their families at this age. At around the age of 37 years the risks of a mother having a baby with Down's syndrome are high enough for amniocentesis to be offered (examination of the fluid around the baby by taking a sample via a needle inserted into the womb). This procedure is not usually recommended for younger, previously unaffected mothers as the procedure carries a risk of miscarriage of a normal fetus.

Children with Trisomy 21 may have serious heart or gastro-intestinal problems; they may have low immunity, and they usually have some developmental delay. The developmental potential of children with Trisomy 21 is very variable, and programmes with early stimulation and well-designed schooling are showing encouraging results. 'Predictions' of outcome for any individual child are, of course, uncertain and building on that child's abilities is the key to success for any one child and family.

V.H.

4

David

OLIVIA BYARD

If I hadn't felt ill that Monday morning in September, I wouldn't have had David seen by the doctor and he would probably have died that day. I was going for a medical check-up myself, and David, my 5½-month-old baby, had a nasty cold, so I thought I would get him seen while I was at the surgery.

While I was waiting for the doctor I trusted that at least we need not worry about any serious illness. The months of anxiety about him were over, and snotty and grizzly though he might be, he was a bouncy and basically fit baby. He'd been born by Caesarean section two weeks before my fortieth birthday, a carefully planned baby and only child of my second marriage. But the day after his birth we'd been frightened by the news that he had a heart murmur, and for the next three months we had worried and taken him for tests, until we learned with relief that he had a fetal hole that was closing nicely, and was not at all dangerous. Yes, by all means take him to France; relax, enjoy him. We did, and he rode around France in the back of our van, a little king surrounded by his adoring subjects, beaming his toothless pleasure at life. At this point the receptionist called my name, so my reverie ended, and we entered the doctor's office.

Our GPs had been very supportive throughout a difficult pregnancy and we got on well with them. This morning the woman doctor was on duty. She checked me over, listened carefully to David's chest, and then surprised me by suggesting that I take him to be seen at the hospital. I asked her if he had bronchitis and she said cautiously that she could hear some sounds in his chest (I realize now that she was being careful not to panic me) and thought that since he had had a heart murmur he should be listened to by an expert. A letter was written and off we went.

David and I arrived at the hospital, the letter was read, and after a surprisingly short wait we were taken into a cubicle. I had just undressed him at the doctor's request when she turned and asked whether he'd ever been that colour before (his lips were deep plum and he had dark blue shadows around his eyes). I felt myself go cold, and managed to say 'no'.

At that point things happened very quickly. We were taken to a ward, X-rays and blood were taken and David, after three blue attacks, was attached to a life-support machine and given some medicine. Then the cardiologist rushed in, Chris, my husband, arrived, and we all trooped to the echo lab, where an echo was done of David's heart. This is an ultrasound picture of the heart working, and even a layperson can see the heart beating, the picture is so clear. But I was not watching the pictures; I was tearful with worry and listening as the cardiologist pointed out what she saw to the registrars. At one point she called out 'it's not something we can't fix', and we had to be content with that until the procedure was over and David was removed back to intensive care.

Then we were asked to go into the cardiologist's office, and there we learned for the first time what we were facing. We sat and listened, Chris looking impassive and me feeling quite sick, while she explained that David had a congenital heart disease called Fallot's tetralogy. There were four things wrong with his heart: a hole between the ventricles, an obstruction, a thickening of the right ventricle, and a narrowing of the pulmonary arteries. He would need two operations to survive, a shunt to provide oxygen until his arteries got bigger and then open bypass surgery to correct the heart.

My first question was how was this possible when David had a clean bill of health from the hospital. What had this to do with the closed fetal hole? She explained that the fetal hole had allowed him to live normally for five months, that it had served as a shunt, and given him the oxygen he needed. Then when it closed, he suddenly went into crisis. It also emerged that the paediatricians had made a mistake, and his last ECG had not been normal for his age, so that they should have been alerted to something much sooner. However, it was too late now for that kind of consideration. We were told that David must have the first operation immediately and that he'd have to go to a referring hospital in London because heart surgery of that kind was not done in this one.

When people first hear that their baby has a congenital heart defect there are certain questions they all seem to ask. First, is it hereditary? No, it is not; it is random in the population. Secondly, was it something I ate, drank, smoked in pregnancy? Again, the answer is 'no'. Three in ten thousand babies have this defect; no one knows why, and until a few years ago it meant an early death. Thirdly and fourthly, what were David's chances of surviving the operations, and what sort of quality of life would he have afterwards? We were told that the chances of surviving the shunt were nearly 100 per cent, the chances of not surviving open heart surgery were up to 18 per cent, and that he would have a good quality of life if he survived both operations.

Then the cardiologist went off to phone the referring hospital, and Chris and I, shocked and tired, went to the hospital canteen for supper and to make plans. There were suddenly many things to do. We were going to London with David, and that involved some organization; yet one of us had to stay with him all the time. We arranged for Michael, my older boy, to stay with a friend, arranged for another friend to take the dog, spoke to Chris's boss and arranged leave, and then made a list of things we'd need in London, and Chris went off to collect them.

Meanwhile I sat with David, watching his monitors and his tiny blue face and fingernails, and answered the endless bureaucratic questions necessary when a child is admitted to hospital. I also described David's regime to the staff, and was given a room to sleep in. Later, Chris brought Michael up to say goodbye. The poor lad was visibly distressed by David's wires and drips. I promised I'd phone him every day and he went off wishing he were either older, or much younger, (he was 14), sure that either change would make it easier for him to cope.

As I climbed into my bed for what was to be a sleepless night,

I reflected that old or young, none of us had any power in this situation; we had no choices. If we were lucky we'd have a live son at the end; thinking about the alternative was unbearable and all too easy. He seemed too small to survive open heart surgery, his heart was minute anyway. And so it went on, thoughts scrambling around like rats in a cage, all night long.

The following morning was fine and clear, the first of three and a half weeks of perfect Indian summer weather, the sort of wonderful settled weather Britain throws at us now and then as a consolation prize for our ruined holidays and damp picnics. David left early in his own life-support ambulance with a doctor and nurse in attendance. The medical staff were happier with his monitors this morning; he appeared slightly less blue and had a little energy, as though he were not struggling for breath all the time. However, they were taking no chances. They felt he should have the shunt urgently, and got me to sign the consent form before he departed, so that staff in London need not wait for our arrival.

Chris and I followed the ambulance half an hour later, arrived at the collection of Victorian buildings in London which is the referring hospital, parked, and dashed into the intensive care unit, an amazing place of beds with little bodies on them attached to ventilators and drips, with a nurse at the end of each one. There we met a most bathotic sight.

In the middle of the room in a tiny cot (the hospital thought they were getting a 5-week-old baby) sat a happy David, holding court to a group of admiring nurses. Since we had expected the drama of an operation, we were stunned. He was still bluish, but compared to the desperately ill children around him, he looked the picture of health. And matters got more absurd immediately. There were no nappies of David's size to be had anywhere in the hospital. David performed while sitting on Chris's lap, and a nurse had to be sent out to a local shop to buy some nappies to make him presentable again.

We were confused. David was dangerously ill but he had stabilized temporarily on his medicine. We were in London, and had no idea when his first operation would take place. Everyone was very busy and we didn't like to bother them with questions. But after a while the routine was explained to us. We were directed to the accommodation officer, allocated beds in the parents' annexe, and given tickets for the staff canteen. Meanwhile David was given a colour echo test to reconfirm the diagnosis of his condition, formally admitted, and taken down to the well-known ward for heart children. Life in London began.

Chris returned home next morning because we had no idea when the operation would take place. I discovered I had arrived just in time for a visit by Princess Diana, a wonderful diversion from worry and anxiety and great fun for the older children on the ward, but I must admit that half an hour after she had left I was so continuously worried about David that I had forgotten she had ever been. A diversion is welcome, but it's not a compensation.

The day after that the doctors did a catheterization of David's heart, a procedure which allows them to insert a probe up through one of the large veins to look at the inside of the heart. They wanted to do this because the surgeon, after looking at the echo pictures of David's heart, thought it might be possible to do the whole corrective operation, the open heart surgery, immediately, if his arteries were big enough. But many measurements would have to be run through the computer first. Chris had said he wanted to be present when David was given an anaesthetic, so I phoned and he left work immediately.

He arrived in time to see David return from the operating theatre. We had been warned that he might look pale because of the contrast medium they use, and he did—white, with bluish bits around the eyes and mouth. He also had to remain on oxygen for three hours. It was a worrying day, not helped by the fact that I had developed cystitis and had to see a local doctor immediately after catheterization. We had to wait over the weekend for the results to be run through the computer, assessed, and discussed by the surgical and medical staff at their Monday morning conference.

I haven't yet described the ward or the area of London the hospital was in. The ward was an old Victorian edifice with high ceilings and eccentric heating. In the baby's room with the sun beating down it was a sweltering 85–90°. Each room had a nurse in it, although, as I learned, there was such a shortage of nurses that they often had to use agency nurses to fill the gaps. The lack of staff had a serious effect on us. The children were all very ill and most of them were waiting for major surgery, which often had to be delayed because of staff shortages. This was frustrating for the nursing sisters and the surgical teams, as well as for the parents.

The nurses explained that they could not afford to live in London even though the work was exciting; wages were low and rents very high. It made sense to train in London and then go and live in the provinces; the work might not be quite so interesting but it was much cheaper to live outside the capital. The hospital never used agency nurses in the Intensive Care Unit, so if staff were ill up there and there were no replacements operations could not be done. The policy made sense, because it was deemed too risky for agency nurses (who were often working overtime) to look after children on ventilators. However, it was infuriating for waiting parents who knew that surgeons and theatres were free, to realize that life-saving operations were being postponed due to lack of nurses and for no other reason.

We were staying in an area of expensive flats and private gardens. These gardens became a source of irritation to me the longer I stayed in London. I needed a garden, felt that Hyde Park was too far to go when I was taking a break from David, and found beautiful, but locked, private gardens everywhere. I finally found a few quiet benches under trees in a corner of the hospital car park, but it seemed so unfair that worried mothers and convalescing patients should have to sit in a car park while the whole area abounded with gardens.

On Monday afternoon the medical team came to see us. The news was good. The new heart measurements had shown that David was large enough and fit enough for them to try the corrective operation in one go. (I learned later that as a result of David's case it is now recommended to take measurements twice, before and after the obstruction has been relaxed by the medicine, because the difference in size of the arteries to the lungs is quite startling.) The surgeons were planning to do open heart surgery on him that Wednesday or Friday.

We received that information in a fairly punch-drunk fashion.

We were glad there was only to be one operation, since he had to have the corrective surgery anyway one day, but this was very final news. He might be all right, but he might also be dead in a few days and we'd have lost him forever. It was hard to confront that possibility immediately. The next few days made it harder.

A couple of months previously I had heard on the news that two London hospitals were closing their doors to emergencies. Like most British people I sighed about further closures and didn't think that it would effect me particularly. But it did. Our hospital was the only referral hospital in London taking emergency admissions. The surgical team may have thought they'd operate on Wednesday, but by then they were chock-a-block with dying babies from all over the region and there was no chance of an operation. One night in that week I was told that they were waiting for a child to die for the only ventilator in London to become free. Furthermore, two more children from the ward died which meant that the nurses were sad as well as pressured, and parents began to panic. There was another child on the ward who was due to have his operation just before David. He had been listed for first on Wednesday; he was now listed for second on Friday. Ten minutes before he was due to go to theatre a critical case was brought in, and they cancelled this child's operation. The father was so upset he could not stop crying.

Needless to say, David's operation was cancelled again and again. The poor surgeon could do nothing but plan to operate the following Tuesday and explain that he had no choice. We all understood that he had to operate to stop babies dying, but it was hell to watch our babies getting bluer and their operations receding into the distance as each new emergency came in. And if the staff waited long enough for David to become an emergency again, which could happen at any time, they might not have time to do the complete repair job but might have to dive in with a shunt just to save his life.

We were all living extremes of anxiety. The nurses were overworked and overwrought, having to choose the bluest babies for operations when all the babies needed operations. They were dealing with anxious parents and the parents of dead children. The parents were miserable and staff was short, so we were expected to spend even more time in the ward caring for our babies. Chris went back to work; Tuesday seemed a long time away and who knew what emergency might come up meanwhile.

To make matters worse, a woman appeared who made my life miserable all week. One learns quickly in a hospital there are parents who are givers and enquire after each other's children, and those who are takers. This woman was the latter type. She went on about what a difficult time *she* had had, and she was oblivious to anyone else's problems. She poisoned the atmosphere of the entire room and gossiped about one parent to another. There was no peace from her, even at night, because she held court in the kitchen of the parents' accommodation and amplified the bush telegraph information about who had died (four children died that week, although only two were on our ward). For four days I endured her all day and all evening and became progressively more drained. To top it off, a young baby was brought in to the bed next to David's and the parents were told within my hearing that the child had no chance of life. They were totally distraught and this dreadful woman was in her element.

Also, our finances were beginning to cave in under the weight of London prices. Although accommodation was cheap, it did cost, and food was expensive. We had eaten out to cheer ourselves up at the beginning of our stay. We soon found that we could not afford to do that, and even meals in the staff canteen for two started to seem expensive. Also, our original packing had been sketchy and we had to provide everything we subsequently needed. Then there were the little presents I bought to amuse David, entertaining Michael and sending money so that his hosts would not be out of pocket, and petrol to and from London for Chris. It all added up. To make matters worse, both our old cars had broken down, and then my glasses broke and had to be replaced at London prices.

I am not religious but I do believe in some sort of collective natural consciousness, and as the days went by I found myself spending more time on the bench in the car park, begging whatever spirits there were in nature to let my son live. It was difficult to imagine 'spirits' of trees and fields and flowers being very interested in such a high tech problem, but I was a mother asking for the life of her child, which could be saved by the hands and skills of other parent's sons and daughters. I could grasp the link back to nature in this fashion and to have the trees listen to my pleas during this time, as they swayed back and forth in the glorious Indian summer weather, gave some sense of peace and considerable strength to carry on. And so, finally, the dreadful second week drew to a close, the ward became more cheerful, and we were optimistic that the operation would take place on Tuesday. The surgeon had personally assured me of this and I believed him.

Chris returned at the weekend and my morale rose. We had been told that in preparation for the operation, as a morale booster, we could take David out for an hour on Sunday into the hospital grounds. We had also been advised to take pictures of him before the operation 'just in case' as they put it. We looked forward to this hour of normality with great enthusiasm and pain, but as it turned out it was a very quick outing. It was soon obvious that David was very ill indeed and we didn't keep him out long. I still have pictures of a peaky-looking child staring solemnly out at a vibrant world, a totally different child from the bouncing little creature who'd held court in France. Now it was very clear that he would have no chance to live at all without his operation; so now we were even more prepared to go ahead.

Chris went home again. He intended to return on Monday evening to be with us before David went down to surgery. David was to be second on Tuesday morning.

But on Monday morning Sister looked worried and evasive. It emerged that they'd cancelled the operation again. It looked as though they'd only be able to do one child on Tuesday and it would have to be the child who'd almost been operated on on Friday. I was miserable; David was going blue very often now and he was deteriorating internally, as his lungs didn't get the oxygen they needed. I understood that the other child took priority but I didn't know how long we could endure this endless wait. When the surgeon arrived and asked me cheerily if I were all ready for the morrow, I had to restrain myself from jumping up and begging him to operate. He was stunned at the news and left the ward quickly. I fed David, did his usual toilet, and then went off and burst into tears. After I phoned Chris, I talked to sister again who stressed that they'd try to fit David in as soon as possible and offered me a couple of days at the hospital in our home city so that I could go home for a few hours. But I decided that I didn't want David transferred anywhere for a day or so. He was too ill and we might miss the only operating slot that became available. Sister and the medical staff agreed that it was the best decision; meanwhile Chris was coming up that evening anyway to lend a little moral support.

After David's lunch I went out for a few hours. I did some chores, sat and read a newspaper in an outdoor cafe, and watched a London apparently full of wealthy, carefree people go by, and I envied them all. But it was good to get out, and I finished my outing on my bench in the car park until I felt able, if not too willing, to carry on with life at the hospital. Then I went back to the ward.

When I arrived back I was informed that David would be operated on the following morning after all, and I sat down winded with shock. From the way sister talked I got the idea that something had happened. A ventilator had become free for David somehow; most probably a child had died to free that ventilator. I was not going to enquire too closely. What was important was that David was being operated on the following morning and Chris didn't even know!

I phoned his workplace but he was on his way to London and couldn't be reached; however, I did manage to advise his colleagues that he would not be back at work the following day. He arrived soon after, absorbed the change of plan, and we prepared ourselves for the pre-operative routine.

In this hospital, parents are taken up to intensive care the night before the operation to see how the children look on ventilators. Each child lay on a bed attached to a ventilator and monitors and a nurse sat at the end of every bed watching each little change on the sensitive gauges. It was explained to us that David would have lines into his body at four places, two in the neck and two in the groin, and that he'd also have a tube down his throat. At that point we were mostly anxious that he should survive to reach intensive care, but it was useful to see the little bodies with their carers, and the anxious parents beside them. They were very still, but they were alive.

Then we talked with the surgical staff, who explained the

operative procedure to us in detail. The house officer said that they would lower David's body temperature to 18° to operate as there was much less risk of damage at that temperature. He then explained how they would connect David to the heart and lung machine, and then how they would repair the damage to the heart by covering the hole with a small patch and, stripping away the obstruction, putting special tucks in it to make sure that it did not grow back. After that they would reconnect David to his heart, warm him up, and try to get it started again—but here he had to give a warning. They sometimes couldn't get the heart to start again. Sometimes it had all been too traumatic for the little heart and in 12 to 18 per cent of the cases the baby died on the operating table. He told us this because they had discovered that the shock was too great for the parents to bear if they were not warned beforehand. What he said made me cry, but the odds were in David's favour, and anyway we didn't have any choice in the matter. This operation was his only chance.

We gave David his last feed that night with special care (he was really very blue now, the slightest exertion made his colour worse) and then we went to bed. I woke in the night and went to the ward to give him his last feed before he was starved for the anaesthetic. It was quiet, and in the gloom with the sleepy sucking baby in my arms I tried to imagine that we were safe at home. The traffic intruded somewhat into my reverie but it was wonderful just sitting holding him, he was such a part of me still.

The next day, 30 September, was yet another glorious day. We were glad because we felt that a continuation of 'David's weather', as we called it, was a good omen. David was due to go down to theatre around 10.00 a.m., so we arrived on the ward at 8 a.m. for his first pre-med injection. This did not make him sleepy and he was not allowed breakfast, so for some while it was a matter of keeping him amused enough not to notice that he was getting hungry. We gave him a bath, dressed him in a minute theatre gown, and after that held him and diverted him until sister felt he could have his main pre-operative injection. Then we relaxed slightly; he didn't fall asleep but was peaceful now, no longer fretting for food, although his clear blue eyes looked puzzled at the way he felt.

I explained matters to him and promised I'd be there on the other side of the operation, until the time came for him to be taken away to theatre. He was still awake and I was worried he'd be frightened, but one of the friendly nurses offered to carry him down for us, as we were not allowed to, and he was carried away in her capable arms quite happily. Then he was gone and we did not know if we would see him alive again.

We had at least five hours to fill while the operation took place, and we had decided we'd go out, even though sister advised me that I might feel the urge to be nearer the hospital and if so, to go to our room. Each parent chose what diversion suited them best, but we wanted fresh air and some peace and quiet, so we drove to Hyde Park, walked beside the water and watched the ducks play.

We sat on the bench and talked. The ducks swam off, but time was passing very slowly (only an hour had limped by), so we wandered over to the cafeteria and ate sandwiches and drank coffee. From a terrace we watched the people, and the very tame birds and wished we were asleep, we were both so tired, and slowly another hour slid by.

And suddenly, there it was, that feeling that sister had warned of. I had to get back to the hospital and fast; there was danger, and I felt needed. So we drove back quickly and went to our room where I lay on the bed, let my tired mind go blank, and didn't so much go to sleep as go into a sort of trance where I was in touch with the operation. And I breathed slowly and listened to my heart beat slowly and visualized David inside me listening to my calm breathing and my regular heartbeat and feeling safe and unafraid. And I knew that they were going to start the heart again and I got Chris to hold my hand. I felt a jolt and a second little heart was beating, just beside mine. It was agitated, but it was beating, and I knew he was alive still. A little later I felt danger again. I didn't know what was happening but I held the agitated little heart tight and soon it all calmed down and became safe again. Time drifted on as I lay there, mentally with my tiny son, and soon I knew the operation was all over.

We had a cup of coffee, and saw that it was 3.30 p.m.. Walking over to the ward I had no worries; I knew he had survived the operation. I could feel him alive. And so he was. The houseman had just come out of the operating theatre and he knew he didn't have to tell us the news. He explained it had been a classic textbook case, and when I interrupted him to ask what the dangerous bit towards the end had been, he said that there had been a few blood-pressure problems but that they had resolved themselves. Then he went off to change.

When we arrived in intensive care, David was lying with tubes in his neck and groin, and a tube down his throat covered in a space blanket; to me he looked dead. I sat down abruptly in the chair provided and tried to take it in. A ventilator was doing all his breathing for him while a monitor gave his internal and toe temperature. The aim was to get the heart working strongly enough so that blood was pumped around quickly enough to bring his peripheral, or toe temperature, up to within one degree of his internal chest temperature. At this point they were very different. Internally he was 38°, or one up on normal, and peripherally he was 27° or very cold, in spite of the space blanket around him. But they were not too worried then, for it was early days yet, so we made sure that he had his little red Ted and pink blanket with him, kissed him, and left quickly to allow the nurses to continue their post-operative monitoring. They liked parents to visit frequently but not to stay too long.

This we did over the next few hours. We made some phone calls to say that David had survived the operation, ate some supper, checked on him now and then, and then both exhausted, went to bed. Thus it was at 5.30 a.m. I found myself awake and dashing across to intensive care, where I arrived just in time. Two beautiful blue eyes opened and looked at me for a moment or two. He was conscious and I was there as I had promised, then he was drugged and drifted off again. I went back and told Chris. We were both elated.

But we were elated too soon. We had thought the worst was over, but the next few days proved us very wrong. During the following day, and for subsequent days, David's toe temperature did not go up, his cardiac output remained marginal, and while the other children recovered, ours lay there totally dependent on the ventilator. So our initial joy became further pain as day followed day and our child got no better.

After two days I returned to my bench and silently screamed to all nature to help. Then I noticed a large flower-bed full of weeds and wondered whether anyone would mind if I tried to set it to rights. A passing official encouraged me to start; and so I did. With sticks and rocks at first, and graduating to a fork and spoon borrowed from the hospital cafeteria, over the next few days I weeded and cleared the entire bed. It seemed as I did that the bed became the heart and lungs of David, and as I gave new energy to the bed to thrive, so I was clearing the decks for David to recover and thrive. And indeed I felt energy flow into him when I went and told his quiet little body what I was doing.

Chris helped me move large rocks and debris, or he sat on a bench and read a book, and so we kept each other company while the struggle for life went on upstairs. The flower-bed soon began to look cared for again; individual plants appeared, and the shape of the design could be seen. Then the hospital flower shop loaned me a watering-can and we started to water twice daily; the shop got me some heathers in different colours and I planted those to shore up the tatty right side of the bed.

Still David lay close to death and still his toe temperature never rose enough. Occasionally it would move a degree or two and they'd remove the space blanket, and then it would go down again, so I'd go back to the garden in misery. (We'd bought him a musical mobile in that first heady morning after the operation, but it was never used. It just stayed silent on his cot, a reminder of how ill he was.) Once I went in and found that they'd removed red Ted and pink blanket. I became very angry so they replaced them quickly. I had read that infants respond to familiar objects even when they are critically ill. I'd already told them that some part of David's brain knew that his favourite things were close to him.

After five days the cardiologist, looking very serious indeed, asked to talk to us. He said that he thought David might have a residual hole and he wanted to do another catheterization to see whether they needed to operate again. We were upset, but had no choice; children were coming and going from intensive care, but our child just lay there. I felt that David's heart would not withstand another operation, but we had to agree to let them try.

So we gave our consent to the procedure and I dashed back to what I now considered to be my garden and nature's description of David's heart. There in the middle was a huge lump of concrete which I'd just left at first weeding because it was hidden from view by a large bush. Now, with Chris's help, I removed it and all other residual debris. Then we went to wait, and as I tried to calm down the tense little traumatized heart that I felt beating just above mine, I became convinced that David would never survive another heart operation; the heart was just too frightened. In fact, I felt increasingly that David's whole being was frightened; it had just been too big an operation for such a young baby and he had gone into retreat, deep inside himself where he couldn't be reached.

We were given the verdict soon enough; there was no residual hole. But the bad news was that there was nothing more that they could do. They had no idea whether he'd ever regain consciousness or whether he'd just linger on until it was time to turn off the machine, a gloomy prognostication.

Something in me snapped. I had to get away for a couple of hours. Chris and I drove to see a friend in North London who fussed over me and gave me cups of tea, and where I generally regained some equilibrium. Calmer, we returned to continue our vigil, and we found an astonishing change. To this day I do not know whether it was the catheterization or removing that lump of concrete that did the trick, but he had turned the corner while we were out. His toe temperature had finally gone up and stayed up, and he was doing a little of his own breathing. It was like a miracle.

After that he got better quickly. By the time his big brother came to see him the following day, the ventilator had been turned right down. In gratitude, with Michael's help, we finished clearing out the area around the garden bed, removed years of debris from the gutters behind the garden and swept away the fallen leaves. Then we ended the afternoon with a truly horrible fast-food meal which Michael thought was wonderful.

David continued to improve. By the sixth day after the operation he was doing his own breathing with the help of a little oxygen and our spirits soared, as slowly but surely, one by one, the various bits of life-support equipment were removed, until they took out his tube and allowed him to wake up that evening. For the first time in a week I was allowed to hold him and try to give him a bottle. It's impossible to describe how I felt holding him after all that time. At that stage a baby is almost part of its mother's body still, and yet due to these circumstances I'd almost forgotten how to hold him. He still had tubes in his neck and groin, and he felt floppy and very weak, but he was alive and was going to live. I was sure of that.

The staff agreed with us. By Tuesday morning we were all ready to leave Intensive Care, and I watched the anguished eyes of parents we left behind. One child had been there for a very long time and there was nothing we could do but send those parents a few flowers (we had been sent flowers by our GP practice the day before the catheterization, and that had lifted our morale incredibly). But we also felt we had looked on the gloomy side long enough. It was now our turn to look forward to recuperation.

The nurses back on the ward were very glad to see David and decreed that what he needed most now was his Mum. The problem was that for me, David seemed more real in the garden than he did in himself. I'd forgotten how to hold him; I'd lost my spontaneity with him; I was frightened I'd hurt him; and, as the nurses made me realize, I was frightened of renewing our physical bond. He had nearly died, and some self-protective part of me felt almost resentful that I should be expected to love wholeheartedly a little character who might, just might, go and die on me. All this is very normal, and the nurses are quite used to this reaction after such a serious operation and a long separation time, but it was important for David's welfare that I should get over this feeling. He needed love to thrive. So on Tuesday and Wednesday while Chris was still there, I divided my time between the garden and David.

I bought and planted several clusters of spring bulbs as a thank you and a promise to the garden that David would thrive, and I said goodbye to all the plants as I watered night and morning. I particularly watered-in the little fir tree that Michael had planted beside the big tree at the centre of the bed.

I learned to hold my son the correct way so as not to hurt his chest and ribs. I held the bottle while he learned to suck again, first slowly and painfully, and later with increased confidence and ability as his throat became less sore. I gazed into his bright blue eyes, smiled, and began to feel better.

Then Chris left for home, and the following morning I didn't have time to water the garden until David had his mid-morning nap, and when I finally went down there I found that someone else had done the watering for me. I was very touched; I was also embarrassed, for I had not realized that others had noticed me working in the garden. Now I knew that other people in the hospital had seen this distraught woman weeding with a fork and spoon I had no more privacy there. The garden was no longer mine; it belonged to the hospital.

That afternoon I took a carefully wrapped David down to see the bed, with its neatly kept rose bushes, little tree, and highland heathers. There seemed little in common between the pale but recuperating baby and the tidied rose bed. But it felt differently; I felt the link in my bones where it had been forged. I said goodbye to the garden and wished it well; it had given me a lot and I would come back to see how it was doing. But life now, for me, had to move on elsewhere.

For suddenly time had run out. It was Friday morning and the transport ambulance arrived much earlier than expected to take us back to our local hospital. After giving presents to the staff, we shuffled along the ward carrying medicines, bottles, baby food, and toys, with no more time for farewells. Soon we drove off, away from the hospital. Then I began to notice the sounds; it was raining; David's weather had finally broken and it was soon pouring. I looked at the grey world outside the ambulance and at the sleeping child in my arms, and we drove out of London, past all the out-skirts, over all the flyovers, towards home.

Postscript

When we arrived at our local hospital, David was suspected of having an infection on the inner surface of the heart. He was kept in hospital for a further two months and treated with antibiotics.

When I heard the news of this further complication I suffered a brief, but acute, nervous breakdown and spent two weeks in hospital myself. Subsequently, I did not stay permanently by his bedside. Hospitals are short-staffed and parents, especially mothers, are encouraged to help. Guilt can stop parents taking even necessary breaks. I had to learn the hard lesson that parental survival is important, too.

Since his operation David has had two infections of the blood, three admissions with high temperatures, grommets inserted twice for recurring deafness, and a short collapse due to scarring activity on the brain, which has since resolved. He has acquired an ENT consultant, a neurologist, and a speech therapist. But otherwise he is happy, active, and doing well. We still worry, especially when he is ill or seems tired; we take minor precautions, but on the whole, we are optimistic, and can even envisage a future now where he has only one consultant, the cardiologist, to see once or twice a year.

He still calls hugs 'gardens'.

DAVID

Fallot's tetralogy is a congenital heart problem consisting of a large defect in the wall between the two pumping chambers of the heart (ventricles), obstruction of the outflow from the right side of the heart to the lungs, right-sided deviation of the vessel which usually leaves the left side of the heart so that it overrides the defect in the central wall, and hypertrophy (over-development) of the right-sided pumping chamber. This group of anomalies leads to insufficient oxygen being carried in the blood, and eventually the child will appear 'blue'. Approximately one in 3600 live births is affected. Some cases present around the time of birth, but usually the diagnosis is made after a heart murmur is heard at a routine baby check.

All children with Fallot's tetralogy need surgery. Sometimes a temporary procedure is needed to allow the child to survive and grow before full correction is attempted. More and more infants are now undergoing successful total correction in one operation.

Survival and long-term outlook is now good for babies treated in major centres.

V.H.

5

Julia

HILARY FREEMAN

Charles and I were in our thirties when we started family life, with well-established careers behind us. Charles read Law and Politics at University and then went on to teach history. I read Sociology, after which I took a course to become a State Registered Nurse. Having staffed for a while I decided to do a further training in psychotherapy, and for several years worked in private practice. At the time I am writing about, Charles was Course Director of a Sixth Form College and writing books on history and politics for sixth formers. I was looking after the children full-time having opted to leave my work until they were much older.

Everything was going so well. We had three happy, healthy children and we had reason to believe our fourth was on the way. We were thrilled.

Then suddenly it all changed. It was seemingly an ordinary Monday morning and we were getting up as usual for work and school. Our youngest child, Julia, who was almost a year old, woke with a cry, so I picked her up, breast-fed her, and all was well again. She sat in our bed playing with a teddy bear when all of a sudden one of her legs began to jerk. She thought it was funny and laughed and her big sister said 'Oh look, Julia's dancing'.

I don't know why, but I knew right then that something was seriously wrong and went straight to ring our GP. He arrived within minutes, by which time Julia had lost her body tone and was twitching in all her limbs. Our doctor advised us to rush Julia to the Casualty Department of our local hospital ten miles away, with a drug at the ready in case Julia began to have a major fit.

The two older children—Barnabas who was six and Isabella who was nearly four, were marvellous—hurriedly dressed, and jumped into the car. Charles drove and I sat in the back with the children, Julia bundled on my knee in her duvet, looking up at me, now and then saying 'Mumum'. Luckily the roads were clear. Had we been half an hour later we would have been caught in the daily monumental traffic jams which bring all approach roads to the city to a near standstill.

A paediatrician saw us almost as soon as we arrived in Casualty. She listened to the brief story of what had happened and then gave Julia a dose of intravenous Valium to try to stop the jerking. Julia then lost eye contact with me but the jerking went on. Charles meanwhile was trying to distract Barnabas and Isabella and to protect them from our mounting anxiety, but their little faces showed that they felt every bit as worried as we did. Once up on the ward it was better for them, with toys and television to amuse them. We met the doctors on duty who told us openly that they did not know what was the matter with Julia, but that they would run some tests to try to find out. Meanwhile the priority was to try to still Julia's jerking. One anti-epileptic drug was given after another but to no avail.

Charles ran Barnabas to school while I rang a neighbour, Penny, to ask if she would collect him at the end of the day. As good fortune would have it, her husband answered and told me that she was on duty where she worked as sister on the children's Intensive Care Unit, just a corridor from where I was. I met Penny as she was coming off duty and it came as a visible shock to her to find that the child she had been hearing about from colleagues during the morning was Julia. It was all so sudden and unexpected; we were all shocked. Penny kindly whisked Isabella away, enticing her with all sorts of exciting-sounding plans and assured us that she would look after her and Barnabas until she heard from us.

It was a relief to know that they were away from the tension on the ward. For the tension was rising. Julia was not responding to any of the medication and her jerking would make it impossible for her to have a brain scan, which was the obvious next investigation. Meanwhile all the blood tests were normal.

By now it was early afternoon and the doctors decided to anaesthetize Julia, as that was the only way to keep her still for the scan.
To be anaesthetized she needed to be transferred to the Intensive
Care Unit, and Charles and I were asked to wait outside. The wait
was agonizing and seemed eternal, but eventually we were allowed
in. There lay Julia, who just hours before had been playing at
home, now attached by tubes and electrodes to an array of bleeping
and flashing machines. It was horrifying to see, but at least she was
at last still and able to rest.

The consultant now called us into his office to put us in the
picture, as much as there was a picture at all. Apparently the
possible diagnoses being considered were a bleed or a viral infection
of the brain tissue, both of which could cause this type of fitting, or
a sudden onset of epilepsy. He sympathized with us for having such
a terrible catastrophe and hoped that the brain scan would clarify
Julia's illness. Charles and I felt stunned. It all seemed so unreal
and so unlikely—yesterday had been such an ordinary Sunday, like
any other, and here we were in another world.

Organizing a brain scan for Julia was enormously complicated.
Not only did she have to be detached from the respirator, monitors,
and drip pumps while portable substitutes were used, but porters,
escorts, and an ambulance had to be arranged coincidentally to
take her to a nearby hospital. At last we were all set and left in a
convoy, ambulance lights flashing. Such hopes rested on this scan.
We all needed something to hang a diagnosis on. The sight of one's
child disappearing headlong into an enormous scanner is awesome.
But it helped to know that Julia was oblivious now to what was
being done to her. A doctor interpreted the scan as we watched.
Julia's brain appeared to be perfectly normal. Was that good or
bad? We assumed it must be good but it still left the jerking
unexplained.

Once back in the Intensive Care Unit, with Julia plugged in again
to the now reassuringly humming and clicking machinery, Charles
and I decided to go back home. We had been reassured that Julia
would not wake up for some days, as it was thought best to keep
her anaesthetized, to rest her and protect her from whatever was
happening.

As we drove home my head spun. Not knowing what lay in store it was difficult to know what to do. First of all we wanted to contact the other children. We called and found them very much at home with Penny, ready for bed, and reading stories. They were happy to stay the night, so we arranged to pick them up before breakfast the next day. Once home we rang close family to let them know what had happened, made some arrangements for Barnabas and Isabella for the next day or two, had something to eat, and went to bed.

The sight of Julia's empty cot opened the floodgates for me and let out all the pain and hurt of the day. The baby I had never been apart from, who should be snuggled in my arms now for a night feed was miles away, seriously ill and nobody knew why. It was almost too much to bear.

Julia remained deeply unconscious for several days, much longer than expected by the doctors, apparently because they could not calculate how long the drug would be stored and remain active in Julia's baby fat. Lying so still for so long she became oedematous and developed pneumonia which, for the first time, made her look very ill. More tests were carried out and more results came back showing nothing abnormal. The pneumonia responded to anti-biotics and physiotherapy and Julia became anaemic, so had to have a blood transfusion. It seemed that one problem was leading to another and that Julia was caught in a downward spiral. So many drips had to be re-sited, we wondered if her veins would cope. Such a mixture of chemicals her body was filled with—what effect would they have? Such were our worries and still there was no clue to the cause of the jerking.

As Julia's birthday came closer it began to look less and less likely that she would surface from the anaesthetic in time for it, yet Barnabas and Isabella were insistent that we should celebrate it in the usual way. So we wrapped presents, made a birthday cake and hoped. Just in time Julia started to stir and began to breathe for herself. She could barely open her eyes, but at least there were signs of life, and on her birthday we were able to hold her on our knees for the first time since it all happened, eleven days before. Barnabas and Isabella decorated her cot with festoons of balloons and birthday cards and invited everyone on the ward to share the birthday cake. In their eyes it was a wonderful party.

The next day, horror of horrors. All of a sudden the jerking in Julia's limbs began again. We were back to square one. The doctors were still no clearer about the cause of the problem. Charles and I were grateful that they were as frank about their bewilderment as they were. At the same time it was frightening and unnerving to see that they were so much in the dark. Several doctors were each giving us their own theory about Julia's fitting and we sometimes came home with differing impressions and expectations. Looking back, maybe it would have been better if they had shared their ideas and given us one view at a time. It was about this time that the possible diagnosis of myoclonic encephalopathy was suggested, and the hope was that if the problem were one of the brain-stem then it might only be physical damage that Julia would suffer, if any at all.

Each day now Julia lightened a little. Charles and I worked out a system whereby one of us could be with her all the time in the hope that our familiar voices might encourage some response from her. Without our friends and neighbours it would have been impossible. Their kindness was immeasurable and with their help with domestic chores we were able to keep home life ticking over. We felt this was vitally important for the other children.

Gradually Julia was able to take fluids through a naso-gastric tube and her body started to function again. Her eyes opened but there was no life in them—no sign that she recognized us except for one brief moment when she said 'Bye bye' to Charles. Maybe, we hoped, it was just the effect of all the drugs. No one could say.

Meanwhile as the numbing effects of the anaesthetic wore off, Julia began to cry. It was a pitiful cry, quite unlike any sound she had made before, and it was obvious to me that she was in pain. Paracetamol helped, but even so Julia was irritable, and although we longed to hold her in our arms to comfort her, moving her only caused more distress. It was a ghastly feeling—so helpless and so unable to give the most basic motherly love. Even though I had kept my milk supply as best I could with the help of the breast pump, when I tried to feed Julia she had forgotten how to suck.

I felt so sad. Sad too because I was losing the pregnancy which had just begun. My upset and anxiety about Julia was too much for it and it was not a fit beginning for a new life. None the less, my sense of loss was enormous, compounded by the fear that I had lost Julia, as I knew her, as well.

A few days later another brain scan was required. This time the journey was much less fraught as Julia was conscious and did not need all the breathing apparatus. We were given a preliminary report of the scan the same day, which again said that Julia's brain appeared to be normal. A recording of electrical activity showed nothing abnormal either, so there was some reason to hope that Julia would recover well.

Meanwhile, though, it was hard to imagine that she might. Julia was completely floppy and inert, her eyes fixed and vacant and her limbs jerking involuntarily from time to time. Four days later, the full report on the scan emerged. Julia's brain showed changes which were consistent with a viral infection. The doctors told us that recovery could continue for months and that it would be a slow business. How Julia would be affected no one could say.

That afternoon Julia was transferred to an ordinary ward where we were settled into a cubicle with room for a put-you-up so that Charles or I could sleep alongside Julia at night. It was good to be away from the highly charged atmosphere of the Intensive Care Unit and to have some privacy, but Julia was not doing well. It was at this point that I reached rock bottom and lost faith in Julia's life. I could not see how such a vulnerable little person could go on like this, and I thought her hold on life seemed so fragile that she would surely die. I could hardly pray. All I could do was to cry.

A few days later we met a new consultant who had been asked to take over Julia's case. She warned us how very serious Julia's condition was and said it was impossible to predict her recovery. She said that she would like to do some further tests for various metabolic disorders which, although very rare, could possibly account for Julia's sudden illness. At the same time she prescribed a drug, not yet used on Julia, to control the jerks and twitches.

To our amazement the drug had almost immediate effect, giving Julia hours of freedom from fits when her arms and legs began to move again, much more naturally. At last we could hold her without causing her more pain and we discovered that Julia perked up to the sound of music, and to Mozart in particular. Then what joy! She began to smile! We brought Barnabas and Isabella in to see Julia more often now and tried to find anything which might give her some pleasure.

Each day we noticed Julia coming back to life a little more and we started to wonder about taking her home. It was four weeks since Julia had been admitted and Isabella was beginning to suffer the strain. It was time we were all home together again. The medical staff agreed and we felt reasonably confident about taking charge of Julia's anti-convulsant therapy.

It was wonderful to have Julia home again even though she was so changed. She had been a contented, bonny little girl, fairly shy with people she did not know but full of fun with us and reaching all her milestones on cue. She was saying a few words, not walking but shuffling about and pulling herself up on the furniture—all just as one might expect of an 11-month-old. Now, four weeks later, Julia could not speak, she had lost all her body tone, and she could barely even focus her eyes on us. We did not know how much her condition was due to the anaesthetic and all the sedatives she had been given or whether this was how she would be permanently.

Suddenly we were on our own and it was strange. Having spent so long in hospital where responsibility for the very life of one's child is automatically handed over to the medical profession, we had grown accustomed to asking for permission and advice. Now Julia was in our hands.

She was still very floppy, with no control of her head and twitching on and off a lot of the time. The twitches were not severe but obvious, affecting different parts. Sometimes her eyes, her face, an arm, or a leg—there seemed no rhyme or reason to them—they came and went at random. Feeding Julia took up a lot of the day. She had lost her chewing and swallowing reflexes so all we could do was to pour pureed food into her mouth, little by little, which took an age. Barnabas and Isabella were very patient, understanding that looking after Julia would take up most of my time for a while. We propped her in a beanbag wherever we were, with all kinds of toys and mobiles strung up to amuse her and to try and catch her attention. At night Julia slept soundly, not twitching at all and looking so peaceful that one could almost believe that it had all been a bad dream.

After a week we kept an appointment with Julia's consultant on the ward where she had stayed. Full of pride in her small achievements we told how Julia had been doing. She was becoming more alert, following us and objects with her eyes, rolling from her back to her side, where she could draw toys to her mouth with her right hand, and she was even attempting to feed herself with a rusk.

We thought Julia was making enormous strides but her consultant did not seem to agree. She listened and then warned us about being too hopeful. 'After all', she said, 'these improvements are very elementary.' We left feeling utterly deflated and dejected, with another appointment for two weeks' time and arrangements for a third brain scan later that week.

We took Julia for the scan. She was very relaxed and not twitching at all, so keeping her still was not the problem it had been before. We did not expect the scan result until our next appointment, as the Easter holidays were upon us.

Charles and I decided that a change of air and scenery would be good for us all. So armed with a referral letter to the local hospital, just in case Julia should take a turn for the worse, we set off for a few days away in the country. Barnabas and Isabella blossomed and we all relaxed and shed some of the anxiety which had built up over the past few weeks.

The weather was gloriously warm that week, so Julia spent a lot of time out in the sunshine, which she seemed to enjoy. Her other great love, we discovered, was water. So each bedtime we gave her a deep, warm bath and all the time she wanted in it. In the water Julia unfurled, giving us beaming smiles of enjoyment. Buoyed up, only her head supported by us, Julia began to move her arms and legs more and more until one evening she kicked and splashed nonstop with great gusto for half an hour. We were amazed. It was wonderful to see such vigour and enthusiasm coming from this little body which had been so limp and inert.

Eating was improving, too, as Julia relearned how to use her tongue and to swallow. She even let us know quite obviously which flavours she preferred. Most exciting of all though, Julia was taking more notice of what was going on around her, Barnabas and Isabella always being the great attraction. We found the extent of their understanding staggering and it was revealing to see how naturally they played with Julia, seeming to know exactly how to make the most of what little movement she had and just what would make her laugh.

The questions the children were asking were the same as ours, 'Will Julia ever get better? Will she ever be able to sit up again?' The fact that nobody knew meant that the answers we gave them were simply, 'we don't know but we hope so'. All along we have been as open as possible with Barnabas and Isabella, explaining as far as we can what is happening. I think what they do is take in what they can cope with at the time and gradually the implications dawn.

A few days after we arrived back home from our holidays, Julia was due to be seen by her consultant again. Charles had to visit his publisher in London that day, so I planned to go by myself, expecting the scan result, but judging by Julia's progress, not unduly worried about it. Just as I was about to leave for the hospital I discovered to my alarm that Charles had left with my car keys. Luckily a neighbour was able to take us and we arrived in time for the appointment.

This time there was no singing of Julia's praises. Obviously the doctor had some news to tell me. Without ado she told me that the scan result was back and she was sorry to tell me that it showed gross damage to the whole of Julia's brain, probably caused by a virus, which would affect Julia both mentally and physically.

I looked at Julia in my arms, the words mentally handicapped ringing in my ears and tears poured from my eyes. Aware that the doctor was telling me about various kinds of help and support available I could not hear a word she was saying and fumbled in my bag for a handkerchief to mop my tears, which I felt were an embarrassment to her. Giving such bad news must be a dreadful task and there can be no painless way of hearing it. I was given another appointment for a month's time and agreed to carry on giving Julia anti-convulsants in the meantime, varying the dose, depending on how twitchy she was.

It was by good fortune that I had no car keys that day. I was too watery-eyed to drive. As I left the main entrance of the hospital I had a stroke of luck. A London taxi drew up, empty, looking for a passenger. I wheeled Julia in, pushchair and all and home we went. I so wished Charles was with us. I would now have to tell him what the doctor had told me and I knew that he would find it hard to take as well. It was not that we were expecting Julia to make a full recovery, we understood that that was not possible. But we were still hoping that if most of the damage had been done to the brain-stem, then even if Julia were physically very disabled, there would still be a chance of some intellectual development. Now we were being told that this would not be possible either—that after what was described as 'such a gross insult to the brain', very little recovery would be likely.

Stark medical predictions made the future look hopeless and gloomy. We now had an enormous change to come to terms with. Every now and then I would wake up in the night with a thud in the pit of my stomach, aware of the words 'brain-damaged child'. But that reaction was more to do with old fears and preconceptions. Although we all worry about the risks of brain damage with certain illnesses and inoculations, I wonder whether one can actually imagine having a brain-damaged child. In abstract it seems like the ultimate disaster. In reality, when it happens maybe it is different. For me it certainly was. Here was Julia: she was still my child and I loved her even more protectively because of what had happened. I was so wrapped up looking after her, however she was, day-to-day, that my preconceptions disappeared and I could only relate to Julia as I had always done before.

Being with Julia was far from depressing. Despite the prognosis hanging over her, she continued to grow stronger, to become more responsive and to relearn some of the skills she had lost. It was a slow business and by no means a steady one. There were days when Julia was twitchy and far away, sleeping much of the time, and others when she was bright-eyed, alert, and full of energy. We tried to discover correlations between bad days and possible causes, but it was difficult to pin-point anything specific.

Our aim with the drugs was to find a balance between giving her so much that she was totally relaxed and floppy, falling asleep all day, and giving her too little to have any effect on the twitches. It was felt that although nothing had been found to stop the twitching altogether, Julia should have a background cover of anti-convulsants just in case she should have a major seizure. Whether or not the little fits Julia was having were more harmful nobody could say for sure, but short of keeping Julia anaesthetized there was no more to be done.

Julia had been in hospital for the month of March. By the end of May she was having regular sessions at home with a teacher coun-sellor and physiotherapist, both of whom we found enormously helpful, with a fund of experience and ideas about how to encour-age Julia's development. She was doing well. One thing she had not lost was the 'will to do' and she certainly had perseverance.

In June we discovered I was pregnant again, and we were de-lighted. We had very much wanted another child and we felt ready to cope. It was important for the whole family that life should go on, to look ahead and not recoil with the shock of what had happened.

During the summer months, Julia's twitches largely subsided, leaving her with a few very brief fits most days. At the same time her tone improved and it was as if we were watching her retrace the steps of her early development but in slow motion. It was wonderful to see. The first time Julia lifted her head up while lying on her front we were speechless with delight, hardly daring to believe it was more than a fluke. And on she went to roll from side to side, to catch her toes and suck them, to pull herself up to sit while we held her hands saying 'Up, up'. She also began to grip well with her right hand and would amuse herself with rattles and bells, seeming to be really excited when she managed to make anything move. Our physiotherapist suggested that we tried sitting Julia in a little wooden corner seat, which we did. In this she could sit holding her head up for half an hour at a time while she knocked toys about on a big tray fixed in front of her. It was a great success.

By September Julia was drawing her knees up underneath herself and then pushing herself forwards by straightening them again. In this way, combined with rolling she was moving about, obviously heading for toys she wanted several feet away. I enrolled Julia in a music class for babies and toddlers and took her once a week to enjoy the singing and wonderful array of sounds. Another high spot of the week for her was a swimming session with a group of children from our local special school, and there she discovered the joy of standing on her feet with lots of support. It was always Julia's enjoyment of life which made all the hours and hours of exercising spent with her so rewarding and worthwhile.

Patient though they were, Barnabas and Isabella did not always see it that way. Understandably, they sometimes complained about the number of people who came to see Julia and about how everyone always wanted to talk about her. Both of them suffered a big knock to their confidence. It must have been as though the bottom had fallen out of their world. We tried to make sure that their lives were full and happy too, and that they each had their own special times with us. But the fact of the matter was that Julia's needs often did have to come first, and feeding her always took up extra meal-time. Hopefully, no lasting damage has been done.

In October Julia had a thorough assessment, when all of the professionals involved with her met to pool their findings and everything about her was tested. After many meetings during the week Charles and I came away feeling greatly encouraged to find how well all Julia's efforts were appreciated. Until then I think we felt that, through medical eyes, Julia was obscured by her bleak prognosis. Now, despite it, Julia was being seen as herself but with enormous problems to cope with.

Christmas came and went and still Julia did well. She was making new sounds, enjoying all the movement she had and seeming to be growing more robust all the time.

Then as suddenly as at first, it happened again. Julia developed a constant jerk which affected her head and one arm. After a few days of keeping a close eye on her, our GP felt that she should be seen at the hospital. So once again Julia was admitted to the ward we knew so well. By now I was 34 weeks pregnant—well, but feeling somewhat cumbersome. I found the prospect of going through it all again daunting and the upheaval seemed tremendous. But there was no choice really, and we felt we must go along with medical advice.

Once again we made arrangements for Barnabas and Isabella to be looked after when they came home from school. Charles managed to get away from work and we drove Julia to the hospital. Disheartening though it was, being back on the ward was not as alarming as our first encounter had been. This time there was a possible cause of Julia's jerking. The doctors thought it likely that she had become tolerant of her medication or outgrown the dose. So the plan was to stop that drug for a week or so while she would be given another anti-convulsant to control the jerks, after which the original drug might well work again. It sounded reasonable. So up went the drip for various drugs to be tried. Just as before, although she became drowsy, Julia went on jerking. It began to feel as though we were on the old track.

This time Charles and I decided not to stay overnight, as Julia was in the habit of sleeping soundly. But we did want to be with her as much as possible during the day. With both of the other children at school now it was easier to do that, with me spending the middle part of the day with her and Charles being there after school and for her bedtime.

Days went by and no improvement could be seen. In fact it was quite the reverse. Julia caught a tummy bug which seemed to be doing the rounds and she began to look quite poorly. Very sedated by the drugs she became even more floppy, but still she jerked. As the dose was increased there was a danger that she might run into respiratory problems, so the doctors wondered about transferring her into the Intensive Care Unit where the equipment was on hand just in case.

Now I really did begin to panic. It felt like a nightmarish re-run of events nearly a year ago. The last time Julia had been put into a deep sleep she had emerged like a zombie. I did not know whether I could bear that to happen again. All I wanted to do was to hold Julia and let time do its healing. Meanwhile Julia's consultant was advising me to stay at home and rest for the good of the baby. That was just what I could not do, and knowing that I was going against medical advice made me feel guilty for following all my maternal instincts.

Julia was taken to Intensive Care. There she slept soundly, luckily with no breathing troubles that a little physiotherapy and suction could not remedy, until it was decided it was time to start her usual drug again. As she came to, Julia was very subdued, but she did not have that empty stare that we had feared she might. What a relief that was! As she was weaned off intravenous food, Julia started to eat and drink again and little by little she began to respond to us, but the jerking went on.

Julia's consultant decided to take some of her blood to repeat some of the tests she had done before. Once again the question of Julia's diagnosis was opened up. She had had another scan which showed no change in her brain. So it still looked probable that the original damage had been caused by a virus. But her doctor wanted to be sure that there was not some other metabolic cause. The implications for the baby I was carrying hung as a grey cloud over me even though I knew that the chance of Julia having an inherited disorder were slim. The test results, we were told, would take weeks to come, so we tried not to dwell on them.

At last, after two weeks, Julia was discharged, back on her original drugs and still jerking. It seemed that the whole episode had been pointless. Just as before it was wonderful to be home and all together once more. But not for long. Two weeks before term I went into labour, not surprisingly as all our babies had arrived early. With special arrangements for Julia to be looked after and a babysitter at home for Barnabas and Isabella, Charles and I left for the labour ward where I gave birth to another son, Thomas. While I was in hospital with him Julia's test results came through and were negative. Another hurdle over—Thomas was in the clear!

It felt so right having another baby. Although our days were busier, Julia's special needs fitted into family life quite naturally, and it seemed healthier that she was not always the focus of everyone's attention. As time went by it became obvious that Julia was not picking up again even though the jerks did settle down. She had clearly suffered a major set-back and was near enough back to square one physically, with very little voluntary movement at all. Even her bowels had stopped working by themselves.

However, remarkable though it seemed, Julia was just the same, with her obvious loves and dislikes, still making the most of everything and enjoying life to her full. She still laughed at the same favourite nursery rhymes and she still came alive to the sounds of Mozart. Knowing very little about music therapy I wonder whether there is something particular about Mozart's rhythms and harmonies which helps to organize a disorganized brain.

While Thomas was newborn, Charles took Julia swimming, and every bedtime she still loved a deep bath with Isabella and Barnabas. I had wondered whether Thomas might oust Julia from their affections. But far from it. Their love and protective feelings for her seem to grow.

When Thomas was a few weeks old we took Julia back to the hospital for an appointment with her consultant. Her conclusion about what happened to Julia was that she had suffered the kind of attack which for inexplicable reasons happens once a brain has been damaged as Julia's was. She suggested trying a different drug which was newly on the market and also made arrangements for another meeting at the assessment centre sometime soon.

We had long planned to move to another part of the country, back to where Charles had grown up, and our moving time was drawing near. So it seemed to be a good idea to have an up-to-date record of Julia's progress to act as her introduction to new Health and Education Authorities.

The meeting was potentially depressing, since it was plain to see that Julia had regressed. But it was not. The paediatrician we talked to had known us in hospital when Julia was first ill, and his main concern was to ease the transfer of Julia's medical care. He felt that there were some things we might like to talk over with him rather than being faced with sudden decisions with doctors we did not know. Very sensitively he brought up the possibility of Julia having repeated attacks which could set her back still further. He asked about our views on resuscitation should Julia ever become that ill and we talked about her possibly dying while still very young.

Far from seeming morbid, it was a relief to have a doctor talk to us in this way, wanting to know our feelings and attitudes. Until then there had sadly been a definite divide, with the medical profession giving us bare facts and friends and relations doing the listening and talking about it all, with our hospital social worker attempting to bridge the gap. Communication was difficult and less of the formality between doctor and patient in hospital would have been a great comfort.

By the time we were ready to move in the June after the February when Thomas was born, Julia was in a pattern of having good days and off days. We adapted, gradually feeling less anxious about her fitting and all the more appreciative of her better times. It was about then that we started taking Julia to a homeopathic doctor in London on the recommendation of a friend. He prescribed some remedies which seemed to help her to weather the ups and downs.

Soon after our move Julia hit another bad patch, but this time we sat tight, nursing her through with valium to relax her during the worst of the fits, taking it in turns to hold her when she was distressed. We very much wanted to keep Julia at home this time and, as we hoped, in time the fitting subsided and she came through smiling yet again. That was nearly a year ago now, since when Julia has been on a much more even keel. Whether the anti-convulsant is helping or the homeopathic remedies keep her stable or if it is just the way she is, we will never know.

There is no doubt at all that Julia enjoys her life. Nor is there any doubt about the enormous gifts she brings to us and everyone who knows her. Of course, it is sad to think of all the joys of life she will not know, and there is no pretending that our life is not difficult sometimes because of Julia's problems. Lifting a three-year-old who is long for her age and no small weight, but who is floppier than a newborn baby is not easy, and every outing has to be carefully planned. But looking after Julia has become so much second nature to us that it is hard to imagine our family life any other way.

We have been very fortunate in finding ourselves in an area where children like Julia are well provided for. She has a busy week with three mornings at a special playgroup, a whole day at school, and fortnightly hydrotherapy. We have met nothing but kindness and offers of help. During the first year after Julia's illness I found it difficult to leave her with anyone else, preferring to look after her myself. But after her relapse I recognized the dangers of such closeness, and then began to appreciate the advantages of sharing her care and having some time when I did not feel so responsible.

One of the problems of caring for a handicapped child is that there is always the feeling that one could be doing more for her, which can result in a permanent sense of guilt. The answer, I feel sure, is to share the care, and that is the solution for us.

So, here we are with a child who in medical and educational language is profoundly handicapped. She can do nothing for herself and has just about no controlled movement at all. She can move her head from side to side to follow people and noises, and with sounds and facial expressions she can indicate when she feels pleasure or distaste. She can smile, laugh, and cry and often makes a variety of sounds in response to being spoken or sung to.

As far as her doctors know the cause of her handicaps was a virulent virus which damaged her brain and left it vulnerable to further damage from epileptic activity.

However, such an objective description says nothing of Julia herself and is not the way we see her day-to-day. As it is, Julia is one of our children who is not growing up like the others. She is a beautiful child with a lovely, joyful presence. We know that Julia's life expectancy is not so long as it would have been, and the more we learn about brain disease the more we realize how lucky we were that Julia survived. She clearly knows us and the people she sees regularly, and has a little understanding—just how much it is impossible to know, and who would presume to judge?

And how are we changed? Before Julia's illness Charles and I had never known anyone severely handicapped. So it has been an eye-opener. Here I run the risk of sounding clichéd, as it has all been said before—about this kind of experience putting everything else in perspective, about how the little things matter, and how nothing is taken for granted. Certainly our life is more provisional than it might have been, and all our plans are 'God willing'.

People have often asked me whether I feel angry about what has happened and whether I ask 'why us?' The answer is 'no'. I think Charles and I are lucky in that we share an outlook on life, believing that there is a purpose in what happens and wanting to cope with what comes our way. No one ever said that it should be perfect, so why *not* us?

Not long after I finished writing Julia's story, she had a very rare reaction to a drug she was taking and she died. She was so very special to us and we all miss her very much.

JULIA

When a child presents with an illness such as Julia's there are a number of possible causes which need to be considered and looked for during the acute stage of treatment.

Julia's illness was eventually presumed to have followed a viral infection affecting the central nervous system. A particular virus was not identified, and this is often the case. A severe illness such as described here usually carries a poor prognosis. The exact nature of disability cannot be predicted for an individual child but may include all degrees of physical and mental handicap.

V.H.

6

Gavin

PAULINE HALLAM

Setting the scene

On 1 August this year whilst on holiday in Spain we celebrated the fifteenth birthday of our eldest son Gavin. Not a very memorable occasion you may be thinking, but for us another real landmark. Let me take you back two years to the beginning of September 1986. Life was seemingly normal enough: my husband Peter travelling from our Buckinghamshire home to work in London and Sussex; Gavin, aged 13, just starting his second year at grammar school; Simon, his brother, aged 9, attending the local middle school; and me working with children with severe developmental delay. Both boys had slight colds, but so did 50 per cent of their school friends, so no action seemed called for, and school continued. Simon was soon back to normal, but Gavin's irritating cough began to keep him awake at night. Our GP said his chest was clear, so no action needed. The cough developed, still keeping Gavin from sleeping, and often causing him to vomit. Our GP indicated that I was over-anxious, so once again no action.

Gavin was definitely unwell, and becoming lethargic, I presumed from lack of sleep. Some days when he went to school I had to collect him during the day because he was ill. Sleeping became almost impossible, his temperature fluctuated wildly, and he began to cough up large quantities of bright green fluid. Our GP eventually prescribed an antibiotic. After a temporary lull, Gavin became too ill to go to school at all. He was developing boils on his hands, and was finding it difficult to eat or drink. Both Peter and I took time off to stay at home with him. Another visit to the GP—another antibiotic—'bring him back on Monday if you're still worried, and we'll think about a blood test.' I took him back the next day, insisted on having a blood test done privately, and arranged to return to the surgery at 11.00 a.m. the next day for the results.

Throughout all this period, I had never been taken seriously, had occasionally been ridiculed, and began to doubt my own instinctive knowledge that something was very wrong. At one point I even suspected Gavin of glue-sniffing—anything to explain the apparently inexplicable.

Peter took Gavin to the surgery on the morning of Friday, 19 September, and was told that the blood tests revealed a serious blood disorder, probably leukaemia. Gavin was at this stage told only that there was something wrong with his blood, and that further tests were needed.

By 12.20 p.m. Gavin was being admitted to our local hospital. We were all in a state of shock, which made clear thought very difficult, but the consultant paediatrician managed to combine patience with admirable efficiency.

By about 9.00 p.m., Gavin's bone marrow had been tested, he had a lumbar puncture, several blood tests, and was being re-hydrated and given intravenous antibiotics. We now knew for sure that he had acute myeloid leukaemia. Gavin hated the needles, begged to be given tablets instead and cried to go home. I had to find the strength both physical and mental to stop being kind and gentle and talk to him really firmly.

I have to admit that once I realized what the next six months to a year was going to entail, I questioned whether we should even begin treatment. In the hour before Gavin's admission to hospital I had read all I could find about leukaemia. Our medical book was not old, having been published in 1982, yet all it said was 'acute myeloid leukaemia is very rare. Only one person in 40,000 dies from it each year; most sufferers are over 60. There is a low cure rate for the disease, which, if untreated, can be fatal within weeks, sometimes even days.'

Was it fair, I asked, to put Gavin through the misery of months of needles, drugs, surgery, nausea and risk of additional infections, when the prognosis was so poor. He had enjoyed thirteen wonderful years of life, and wouldn't it be kinder to let him die quickly and quietly now rather than during some crisis induced by what was not even a guaranteed cure. Peter felt strongly that, at age 13, Gavin should have a say in his own future and that, however small the possibility of success, Gavin should not have the chance taken away from him even by us.

At the time I agreed, perhaps because I was too shocked and confused to do otherwise, but I became grateful for that decision within a very short space of time.

Peter returned home with Simon, to begin the task of creating some order and normality, whilst explaining just enough of what was happening to answer Simon's questions, without frightening him too much.

Gavin dozed fitfully in a cubicle, and I was generously given use of the doctor's office and telephone, so that I could inform my parents and Peter's mother of developments. These were two of the most difficult phone calls I have ever had to make—to keep control of my own emotions, and help others to come to terms with something so horrific that I could hardly believe it myself. After all, two days ago I had merely been an over-anxious parent!

I stayed in the cubicle with Gavin overnight, and began to learn about the sterile procedures which were to become part of our life. By this time Gavin knew he was to be transferred to a London hospital in the morning. We talked a little—Gavin seemed to pass through the stages of fear and anger quickly, and withdrew within himself for a while. I respected this need to be alone with his thoughts. So far, he knew he had a serious blood disorder, that he would be in hospital at least six weeks, and that he would need more tests. That seemed enough to come to terms with for the moment.

Our journey to London the following morning was almost silent. Gavin was totally lifeless, and didn't seem to mind what was going on. I just functioned automatically. And so the next stage began.

Practical matters

For the moment I'd just like to leave Gavin's story and talk a little
about the purely practical matters which, although insignificant in
relation to what was happening to our son, took on mammoth
proportions.

Peter and I both needed to be at the hospital, but did not want
Simon's life to be totally disrupted. This was where our families
and friends stepped in. My brother-in-law, his wife, and young
baby spent the first week of their 'holiday' at our home with
Simon. Meanwhile my mother arranged to retire from work three
months prematurely, so that she and my father could take over on
a more permanent basis. And so our routine developed. I was
granted indefinite unpaid leave of absence from my job so that
I could spend all week with Gavin. We decided that Peter should
return to a fairly normal work routine as soon as possible. I lived in
at the hospital in London from Monday to Friday, whilst my
parents moved into our home to take care of Simon. Peter worked
Monday to Friday, then took over at the hospital so that I could
return home to spend time with Simon. Peter and I met up at
'handover sessions', and at times of crisis when he was also needed
at the hospital. Obviously not an ideal situation, but it meant that
we both maintained contact with both children. Friends arranged
to ferry me back and forth to the hospital, as I was quite incapable
of driving or coping with public transport in the early days. Soon a
rota was established, and tolerant friends drove in and out of
London for many months—usually with a sleeping passenger. My
weekdays at the hospital were exhausting enough, but since I spent
most of my 'recuperative' weekends on the side-lines at Simon's
football matches, I was no great conversationalist by Monday
morning.
  Emotionally, Simon seemed to cope well with his change in
routine. In retrospect he even says he enjoyed having so many
different people around. The dog was quite another matter! He
really didn't understand what was going on, and took to howling

under my bedroom window at 3.00 a.m. at the weekends. A habit incidentally, which he still retains!

We had no immediate money problems, but obviously we were without my salary for almost seven months, and there are many 'hidden costs' to having a child in hospital.

The specialist hospital

I will now return to Saturday, 20 September, and our arrival at the hospital in London. Nothing I say from here on should be interpreted as a criticism, as we have nothing but praise for everyone involved. However, it is a shock to arrive at such a renowned hospital to discover that there isn't actually a bed to spare. I soon learned that the shuffling around of patients to accommodate newcomers is a common occurrence. After a brief stay in the corridor Gavin was installed in a corner bed, which afforded a little privacy on what was an unbelievably noisy, cramped ward.

Gavin soon stunned me by saying 'I think I must have cancer'. The actress Pat Phoenix had just died from cancer, and he also talked about this. I said that not everyone with cancer dies from it and the doctors were in fact checking the diagnosis of our local hospital before coming to talk to us. They soon arrived and explained everything to Gavin with what was, for me, horrifying honesty. They totally agreed with the diagnosis. The terms leukaemia and cancer were used immediately, and to my surprise Gavin began to ask his usual probing questions. Can you cure me? What is a remission? How long will I have to stay here? If I have a Hickman* catheter will you take this drip out of my arm?

We began to talk about staying in hospital for three months now, so gradually Gavin was beginning to accept this time-scale.

Gavin asked me to read to him. I shall never know why I picked up the book *Jonathan Livingston Seagull* by Richard Bach just before we left home, but it could not have been a better choice. At frequent times during the next few days I would read it aloud whilst Gavin seemed to doze. For those of you who don't know the book, Jonathan is a seagull who breaks all the rules, knowing that

* see glossary

nothing is beyond him. He lives by the precept 'the gull sees farthest who flies highest'. Somehow the message seemed most appropriate.

I couldn't eat for several days. One of the other mothers on the ward took me off to the kitchen and made me have a cup of tea, saying that she understood how I felt, but they'd all gone through the same emotions and had learned to come to terms to some extent for the sake of the children. We still keep in touch, even though her son died whilst Gavin was undergoing treatment. During the following months I tried to 'adopt' some of the mothers of newly diagnosed patients in the same way when they seemed to be walking around in a shell-shocked state. Some very unusual friendships develop on a children's cancer ward. One of the fathers once said to me 'You've joined a very special club now, and although none of us want to belong, we've got to make the best of it.'

We were quickly given books to look at together about Hickman catheters, and another patient came to show us his *in situ*. Gavin and I tried to make ourselves look at the pictures and talk about it but it wasn't easy. Everyone was bald in the pictures, and to our inexperienced eye, Betadine looked just like blood.

Last November one of Gavin's friends was diagnosed as having a tumour in his throat. He is a wonderful artist and drew constantly during his first few days in hospital. All his pictures finished at the ears. The tops of the heads were left open. Perhaps this was his way of dealing with a ward full of bald heads.

Actually, losing his hair did not cause Gavin too much distress. He continued to 'spike-up' his remaining strands to the bitter end and declined offers of wigs, preferring to go out hatless unless the weather was too cold. We even devised a way of getting through the supermarket check-outs quickly. Gavin would remove his hat with a flourish, revealing his bald head and people would disperse rapidly. Fortunately, Gavin's sense of humour remained with him for much of the time.

On Sunday, 21 September 1986, I began to write a daily diary. It helped me to cope with each day, and eventually became an encouraging record of progress. Gavin used to 'send me up' dreadfully, saying it was probably just like the diary of Adrian Mole, but nevertheless I persevered. One year later, on 21 September 1987,

I allowed myself the indulgence of reading it all through again. To me this had been a most therapeutic exercise, helping to put my thoughts in order, and providing me with some concrete memories of a son who might well have died at any moment.

The diagnosis of cancer does, of course, still sound like a death sentence, and it is only after becoming so closely involved that anyone can begin to be in the least bit optimistic. Peter and I both certainly believed Gavin was going to die very soon, and I had even planned his funeral along the lines of a celebration of his life. I have spoken to other mothers whose first reaction was just the same.

It was difficult to get other people to use the taboo words cancer and leukaemia openly, but we insisted that there were no pretences. Gavin asked that I should ring his closest friends and say exactly what was wrong, as he did not want there to be wild rumours.

Cards, letters, tapes, etc., arrived for Gavin in a constant stream from teachers, ex-teachers, friends, and relations, and soon his corner of the ward began to look quite acceptable. Gavin commented that all the cards said 'Sorry you're feeling ill' or 'Hope you are better soon' but none had the courage to write 'Sorry to hear you've got cancer'. It then became our policy to create a 'home' for Gavin, and each week we would buy a poster, bring in his clock, or change his pillow case and bedspread to bright colours. Gavin asked for a mirror to monitor the changes in his appearance and, despite protests from our parents, we willingly obliged.

Privacy became very difficult. With a 14-year-old girl in the next bed, and only a glass partition, bedpans and urine bottles became a nightmare for both, but strategically placed posters helped a little.

Noise was another matter. A teenager is not very tolerant of a baby crying at the best of times, but at a time like this it often became unbearable. We bought Gavin a Walkman, and story and music tapes, though we often resented the fact that we couldn't sit in silence or just talk to each other. Gavin joined the ranks of television addicts, with a policy of 'if you can't beat them, join them', and this is a habit we are finding difficult to break even now.

At night, Gavin attempted to sleep with an eye-mask and

ear-plugs. His greatest joy on coming home was to sleep in a pitch-black room, on his own, with the door tightly shut.

Gavin's treatment progressed fairly normally through two DATs and a MAIZE.* The Hickman was a wonderful blessing, and the most traumatic period was when his first Hickman had to be removed and treatment continued through partially collapsed veins in his hands and arms.

He had made friends with the psychologist, and this was when he really came into his own, helping Gavin through relaxation and hypnosis to cope with his fear of needles.

At age 13, Gavin had obviously started to become independent of us to a certain degree, and now, of course, this was taken away from him. We all tried to make light of the situation, but it was not easy. Whenever possible he attended the hospital Youth Club, Scout Group, and Radio Station, but treatments often made this impossible. He continued some basic school-work with the Hospital Teachers and had a few music lessons on an electronic keyboard. His home computer was installed in the corner, and we tried to fill his days.

We soon felt we were part of the team fighting for Gavin's life, and Gavin continued to ask searching questions of all around him. His friend in the Haematology Department showed him how to take a blood count, his doctor took him off to irradiate blood for one of his friends in a cubicle, the nursing staff showed him their pop concert programmes and continued to administer cytoxic drugs under Gavin's ever-watchful eye. The medical secretary visited daily, with jokes and tricks, and the microbiologist kept us on our toes in her own special way. We felt all were our friends. Gavin began to resent the drowsiness caused by the anti-emetic drugs and finally refused to have them. He said that he had no control over the disease, no control over the treatment, but he was going to remain in control of his mind. The vomiting and diarrhoea just became an accepted part of his routine.

Just before Christmas 1986 he took up a new hobby—photography. This has continued to this day, and he recently won a prize

---

* These initials represent the drugs used in the chemotherapy regime.

in a competition. The ward was compiling a board of named photographs of staff involved with the children. Gavin was entrusted with a polaroid camera, a cork wallboard, and films. It was a great success. At about this time the Christmas flood of celebrities was arriving at the hospital and Gavin made good use of the camera yet again. Gavin designed some Christmas cards, one of which was reproduced by a marketing organization. He later adapted this design for the cover of the hospital's own book for new patients.

We spent Christmas in hospital with anyone else too sick to get home. We had a wonderful time; one of our best Christmases ever. Drip stands were festooned with streamers and balloons, fancy dress was the order of the day, and many off-duty staff arrived for the celebrations. I shall always remember the incongruousness of one sister dressed as a giant bumble-bee, administering drugs to a sick but happy child.

Eating was obviously one very big problem. Not only is there sickness and diarrhoea but also mouth ulcers. Early on we watched other mothers enticing their offspring for hours on end. We quickly came to an arrangement. When Gavin felt well enough he would eat, as he knew it was important, but we were not to become totally preoccupied with food. This seemed to work. After one lengthy non-eating session Gavin asked for a packet of pickled onion flavoured crisps. Needless to say they were totally unsuitable and were quickly returned! Each little trip home between treatments was invaluable as it gave us all a chance to play at being a normal family again, and to build up resources to face the next session. However, the returns were sometimes rather traumatic, as was Hickman care at home without the expert advice of Sister Sue on hand.

By February 1987 Gavin had completed his initial course of chemotherapy, two DATs and a MAIZE. There had been many traumas on the way, not least when 'Nemo' the Killer Whale at Windsor Safari Park, a long-time favourite of Gavin's, died of cancer of the bone marrow.

Gavin now discussed the options for continued treatment with everyone he could, and then declared that there was no way he could cope with repeating all three treatments all over again. He was anxious about the periods of susceptibility to infection and falling blood counts and did not want to spend another five months in hospital. He requested the alternative treatment of one dose of melphalan and then wanted to get on with his life again. His wishes were respected and we all returned home on 6 March with treatment complete. His Hickman was removed on 29 April and we then set about the task of rebuilding our life at home.

From the moment of Gavin's diagnosis we tried to find literature which would help us become familiar with the disease, its treatment, and probable prognosis. We realize that there is no way as yet for doctors to predict which children will survive, but we did need something to cling on to. To read 'the results with other forms of acute leukaemia unfortunately fall far short of those now being achieved with acute lymphoblastic leukaemia (ALL) and "cures" are exceptional', is very negative and depressing. To find acute myeloid leukaemia (AML) dismissed in one short paragraph at the end of a publication leaves much to be desired. We all learnt how to live one day at a time, but it is in our human nature to want to look to the future. As an example, whilst Gavin was so ill, we continued to pay instalments on a school's cruise to Greece, Egypt, and the Holy Land, never quite believing he would actually be allowed to go. In February 1988, with his immune system hopefully able to cope, he really did go, as a normal member of his school party.

Psychologically and educationally Gavin does not seem to have suffered at all. He is repeating the school year he missed, and soon seems to have made new friends. He is a more positive and determined person than before, and his enthusiasm for life is admirable. He did not find hospitalization a totally negative experience. Obviously there were moments of acute depression, but he always managed to talk to someone about it—often the long-suffering nursing staff in the early hours of the morning! He made many friends, and appreciated the 'team effort' that went into his treatment. In spite of many deaths whilst on the ward, he did not find the atmosphere continuously morbid, and every effort was made within restrictions of the situation, to ensure that his quality of life was the best possible.

He has met many celebrities. Some have kept in touch since.

He has visited Paris, Greece, Egypt, Turkey, and Spain. He was nominated for a Child of Achievement award by his school and received a Chief Scout's Award for Meritorious Conduct. He has celebrated two birthdays since diagnosis. We have had two family holidays together. He has been on sponsored walks for Leukaemia Research Foundation. He has been on 24-hour hikes with his scouts. He has been gliding, canoeing, swimming, cycling, and best of all, he feels that he has been accepted back as a normal member of his peer group. He knows that the disease may recur—at the end of treatment he said 'Well I think this deserves at least two years of remission don't you?'

Peter and I feel privileged to have been able to spend so much time in his company. We enjoyed our enforced periods together, escaping with him from the hospital whenever possible to visit shops, museums, exhibitions, parks, etc.

Gavin's last school report said:

A thoughtful and outward-looking approach to life have been the hallmarks of Gavin's contribution. What a joy it is to see him so full of life and fun. Others have a lot to learn from him.

7

Karen

KAREN WOOLLEY

It was 17 March 1988 when I was diagnosed as having leukaemia. I will always remember that day. I was only 15 at the time.

I had been in hospital for two days, but I didn't know what for. I had had a bone-marrow biopsy on the day I was admitted, but it had meant nothing to me. On the Wednesday when my Mum came to visit, she started talking about leukaemia; I cannot remember what it was she said. I sat down and just dismissed it. After all, something like that wouldn't happen to me. Unfortunately it did. No more was said on the subject, then on the Thursday afternoon, my doctor came in and said he wanted to talk to my parents and me and did I want to be with them or would it be best to talk to them first. I left it up to him. At 4.00 p.m. my Dad arrived to pick me up, so he thought. He had been given a message to pick me up and that everything was fine. When he arrived I was having a blood transfusion. I was so anaemic I was almost transparent. My arm was like a balloon from a previous blood test, and as for the rest of my body, I looked as if I had been in a punch-up, I had so many bruises.

When the doctor arrived, he took my parents into the office with a couple of other doctors and the ward sister.

A little later, the doctor and sister arrived carrying a tray of tea. They looked so serious. Both of them sat down and the sister explained to me that what the doctor was about to say was very important and that I should try to understand. I knew it must be serious.

The sister took hold of my hand and the doctor started to explain things to me. He told me that I had leukaemia. I didn't know what it was or where it came from, I just know that I had 'it'. He explained that I would have to undergo special treatment and that I would lose all my hair. I would have to take drugs for quite a while. Who said it would be easy?

One thing that will always stick in my mind for the rest of my life, is the tears in my parents' eyes as they entered my room after being told what was wrong with me. I just wanted to cling to them, to reassure them that I was going to be all right. I had God with me, and each day I had the assurance that no matter what was going to happen to me, God would always be there to take away all the misery.

On the Friday I had a Hickman line* fitted down in theatre, I also had my first lumbar puncture†—one of many. From then onwards it was various types of chemotherapy (which made me lose my hair) then radiotherapy, lumbar punctures, and bone-marrow biopsies.

My immune system was pretty low, so I had to stay in my room, 24 hours a day, for 7 weeks. I was allowed home for one weekend, but had to be back early on the Monday for my second bout of chemotherapy. It was hell. For one week all I did was vomit. The thought of food made me feel so sick.

My Mum was with me constantly, and every free moment my Dad had, he was also with me. Every time I saw them, I hurt inside, for their faces were filled with so much sadness.

After my second dose of chemotherapy, my hair fell out. I kept getting asked to have a wig made. I refused, as I was more worried about it falling off.

I will always remember the mask I had made, ready for my radiotherapy. I felt like I was suffocating under the pastry like covering which was being moulded over my face. I only had a tiny hole to breathe through, everything was pitch black.

Since my radiotherapy, life hasn't been easy, but it has been easier.

* A line giving direct access to the venous system for drug administration and blood sampling.
† Insertion of a needle to take a sample of the fluid from around the spinal cord.

I know that I will be on drugs, and have to have vincristine injections for a long time, but I know that at the end there will be a rainbow, and if I had to undergo all the treatment again, I would, just for the love of my family and life.

Often when I am on certain drugs, I get very depressed and moody, I know it is hard on my family, but I just can't help it. Living with a leukaemia patient is hard going. Everybody tries to understand. I know this will sound harsh, but people don't really know how you feel unless they actually experience it. God forbid. I wouldn't wish leukaemia on anybody, not even my worst enemy.

The love and support which I have received from my family, my pastor at Church, and the doctors, helped me a lot, they helped me to pull through.

8

David

DAVID GIBSON

My time in hospital

I was first diagnosed as having leukaemia in January 1988, when I was 13 years old. At first when my doctor explained what was wrong with me, I wasn't too worried because I didn't know very much about my illness. Also, my doctor had said it was curable, so I automatically thought I was going to be all right. But about a fortnight into my treatment I was starting to feel very depressed and wondering if I really was going to be OK. At one point I really thought I wasn't going to make it, and I wanted to end it all. But, gradually, I got to know the doctors and nurses, and they explained everything that was going to happen piece-by-piece. Eventually I thought, I have to think positively or I am not going to make it. That is now my motto, although sometimes it does become very difficult, because at times when I am having treatment I feel very ill and ALONE. It really helps if you have someone to talk to all the time, but because my Mum has to work I feel very lonely, and that is when I feel the worst. Everyone is really great at the hospital and they try to come and talk to me, but they are very busy sometimes.

When I got home after my first bout of treatment I went straight up to my room, lay on my bed, and started crying. I really don't know why I did this. I suppose it was just relief at being home again.

After this, I went into hospital three or four times, for a fortnight at a time. These visits were easier because they were short compared to the first lot. Straight after these I had to have radiotherapy. This was very scary because all of a sudden you were alone in a big area lying flat on a table with a massive machine behind you. I shudder to think how younger children felt about this.

In May 1988, I received a letter from my doctor saying I was in remission. I was ecstatic! I was in remission until December 1988, until on a routine visit to the clinic my doctor said that he wanted to check my bone marrow. After the operation my doctor came and told my Mum and I that I had relapsed. I was distraught! All I could think of was that I would have to go through everything all over again. The doctor said I would need a bone-marrow transplant, so eventually he took blood tests from my family. Fortunately my brother is a perfect match. I have just had a new kind of treatment for which I was in hospital for six weeks. I found it really hard going. Being my age in a children's hospital isn't easy but it is better than being in an adult hospital. Also all the staff treat me like a young adult which is good. In a month I am going into hospital for more treatment before my bone-marrow transplant. I feel as if just as I get used to being at home again I have to go back into hospital.

Hopefully after all this is over I can get back to normal again. It is quite funny watching young children's faces when they realize that I haven't got any hair. I used to get really upset about this but now I just laugh about it. I hope in ten years time I can look back at this time in my life and laugh about it too. But at the moment I don't think it's very funny.

David Gibson died in November 1989, aged 15, eight months after this was written. He was a fine young man. Those of us who knew David will always remember.

V.H.

GAVIN, KAREN, AND DAVID

Leukaemia is the commonest type of malignant disease in childhood. It affects white blood cells, which are usually involved in protecting the body from infection. Proliferation of malignant white cells depresses the production of normal constituents of the blood.

There are different types of leukaemia both in children and in adults. Acute lymphoblastic leukaemia (ALL) is the most common in childhood, accounting for 75–80 per cent. Other acute leukaemias, including acute myeloid leukaemia (AML) account for a further 20 per cent. The incidence of leukaemia in childhood is about one in 2000 children. Without treatment it is usually fatal. Treatment involves long and aggressive schedules with chemotherapy and radiotherapy. During treatment, children must attend hospital frequently, and suppression of normal bone-marrow function increases the children's risk of infection and bleeding.

Prognosis varies with the age and sex of the child, the type of leukaemia, the white-cell count at diagnosis, and evidence of widespread involvement.

In the last twenty years, prognosis has improved dramatically—more than 50 per cent of children with ALL now become long-term survivors.

Other types of childhood leukaemia have proved more difficult to treat. Bone-marrow transplantation, however, is likely to become of increasing importance in the treatment of children with leukaemia who do not do well on initial standard treatment, and it seems probable that survival rates will continue to increase.

V.H.

9

Richard

SHIRLEY EVELEIGH

My diary entry for 20 September 1987, reads: 'I had a son and his name was Richard. Visitors this evening brought photographs of the flowers on his grave. They were very beautiful but is that all there is left of Richard? I don't believe it. Richard who was never still, who loved to be out in the garden, especially playing cricket and who had little time for television except for SuperTed, his favourite cartoon. Richard was the one who would walk or cycle with me in the countryside he loved. Where was my soulmate? I look at his photograph and turn around expecting to see him there. I have spent this week looking for Richard. I walked down the lane to the farmyard and climbed up the steep field, looking back down at the pond as we used to a year ago. I have been on all our favourite walks, sometimes crying out 'Where are you, Richard?' But then I left the steep field and crossed the road to the churchyard. I didn't find Richard there either, only his shell is there, the earthly body he no longer needs.'

Richard's story begins on 14 March 1985, when I met him from school to find he had a huge, badly swollen, black eye. He had collided with a small girl in the playground. That black eye was not to disappear for months, but it was of no great concern as memorable black eyes come to mind when he was a toddler. If I had known then what I do now—but I was to say those words repeatedly over the next eighteen months.

Towards the end of the autumn term Richard's teacher and others commented that he was not as lively as usual. He seemed to be very quiet and was particularly fussy about food. He had often had periods of not sleeping in the evenings so this, too, was barely commented on.

After Christmas, Richard frequently complained of earache, so I took him to the surgery. He looked very pale to me, but I suppose a stranger might think he was a naturally pale child. Our own GP was away and the new man declared there was nothing wrong with Richard; no infection, probably catarrh, so I was despatched home with a bottle of medicine. I calmly accepted that, as I did the same man's reticence to pay a home visit when both children were ill with high temperatures a fortnight later. Richard had earache then and I was advised, on the telephone, to give him Disprin. What damage I could have done!

I have since asked myself why wasn't I more persistent; why did I believe he must be right—he's a doctor? I think because I came from a generation whose parents held doctors in awe and their word sacrosanct. Too late I have learnt that they, too, are human.

I will never forget Sunday, 16 March. It was the last day of Richard's life when we were all happy. Happy in our ignorance that there was nothing really wrong. We walked in the RSPB reserve in the Forest of Dean, I carrying Richard most of the way as he tired easily.

The following day I took Richard to the surgery, where I was relieved to find our own GP back. Two days later Richard, hugging SuperTed, his favourite toy, was admitted to the Children's Ward of our local hospital and given a room in the Oncology Wing where the leukaemia patients were treated. A brass plaque at the end of the corridor showed that the unit was mainly built with generous contributions from the Cancer and Leukaemia in Childhood Trust. I had never heard of it until then but I was to meet some wonderful people involved with the Trust. The rooms were very bright and everything looked new, Richard's room overlooking the garden complete with bird-table and Wendy House.

We were questioned by a number of doctors and nurses, and I was told they would be looking for leukaemia. I had not slept the previous night because that very word had been constantly on my mind as Richard lay beside me in restless slumber. Whilst Richard was under general anaesthetic having a bone-marrow test I wandered around outside sobbing. I didn't understand why my life had suddenly been shattered. This sort of thing doesn't happen to me, I thought. It is always somebody else one reads of in the newspapers, tragedy never involved you!

Back in the ward Richard was fighting an oxygen mask. I shudder now when I see such masks. That night was the first of many spent in a reclining chair beside my son, watching the clock.

The following day we met the doctor who was to become such a friend and ally. Richard definitely did not have leukaemia but aplastic anaemia, for which a bone-marrow transplant was a possibility. I breathed a sigh of relief because I had never heard of that, so it could not be bad.

To think that a week ago Richard had, for the first time, played football for his school, so proud to have been chosen and the youngest in the team. They won, of course. If Richard could do that on a haemoglobin* count of 4, his determination would bring him through this disease and enable him to do anything he wanted.

Richard was discharged temporarily feeling much better for the blood and platelet† transfusions. He was happy because it had been recognized he was ill and something was being done about it. The whole family had various blood tests over the next week and on 27 March Richard was to have another bone-marrow test. This was unfortunate, as he was to be enrolled as a Cub that evening. He had only attended meetings for a few weeks but already it meant a lot to him. That day our son showed the will-power and courage that was to carry on until his hour of death. The consultant told him that if he felt well and was not sick after eating something she would discharge him in time for the meeting. Richard was eating toast an hour and a half after the anaesthetic! I was so proud of him that night, in full uniform for the first time as he was enrolled into the Green Six.

For the next month we lived in a false sense of security with uneventful visits to hospital for transfusions. Our paediatrician had

---

* Haemoglobin: red pigment which carries oxygen in the blood.
† Platelet: blood constituent involved in clotting.

been conferring with a professor at a London hospital who now wanted to see Richard.

The unassuming façade of the specialist hospital revealed an impressive area, although our high spirits were dampened when directed to the consulting room in the basement. The corridors were unclean and the room a windowless box. The professor was positive and full of hope. There was one treatment he wanted to try before a final decision was made. In a few cases a course of steroids had stimulated the bone marrow into natural regeneration. Richard was to take this for a couple of weeks, but if there was no improvement the professor would recommend an immediate transplant, from which there was an 80 per cent plus chance of recovery. There was no need to wait, especially as Rebecca appeared to be such an excellent match; how lucky Richard was to have a sister so perfectly compatible. In this case, none of the drug treatment I had heard about would be suitable and the professor's words 'they will not work' were imprinted on my mind. I was much impressed by this tired-looking but obviously very caring man who proceeded to tell me that he would not be able to help Richard at his Children's Hospital because of a lack of specially trained nurses. Transplant patients needed intensive nursing, and although the facilities were available staff were not. He actually said he was in despair, as Richard was not the first patient he had turned away. We would be referred to another hospital if necessary.

I had heard of cuts in the Health Service, read the odd article, but am ashamed to say had never paid the situation much attention. It is not until one becomes involved that it matters. How blind we are to important issues when they do not affect us personally! Richard could not be treated at the Children's Hospital because of lack of staff! Surely children should be given top priority? This hospital was well-known. How could such a situation be allowed to develop?

When we returned two weeks later the professor had decided Richard should have a bone-marrow transplant. Our son did not have enough good blood to endure delay, and we were to be referred to the next hospital where everything would be put in hand within a month. Tony and I travelled home in silence but not in hopelessness. Richard could, indeed would, be cured. Rebecca greeted the news with tears but, when I explained that she was so special she was the only person in the world who could help Richard to get better, 'I'll do it, Mum' was the speedy answer. How lucky we were to have such a daughter, and she was only 11.

In May 1986, when we first took Richard to that hospital, its entrance hall bore close resemblance to a tube station. It was dirty, unkempt, and literally strewn with litter. The corridors were not much better. We were going from bad to worse.

The consultant calmly informed us that he had decided to try for a course of drug treatment. We were speechless. I tried to tell him the professor had said Richard was an unsuitable case for any type of drug treatment but he did not seem to listen to my words, simply saying that there had been a difference of opinion over the treatment of this patient. He told us not to worry, because we could always fall back on a transplant. We felt he was not honest with us then or at later times. The drug treatment was successful in 50 per cent of cases, and I believe he must have thought Richard stood a good chance of recovery or he would not have risked what he must have known was his life by delaying. Was the delay because he had a shortage of staff as well? Was he using this treatment on patients to try and ease pressure on his scant resources? We will never know the truth, but I do know that Tony and I were confused, upset, and desperately worried. We had taken our son to see an eminent haematologist—one of the country's leading authorities on bone marrow—only to be told by someone else of equal standing in the profession that he recommended an alternative course of treatment. We did not know who to turn to. Who was telling the truth? Richard's very life was at stake and we both felt impotent. I think, on reflection, that we made our greatest mistake by not causing a fuss and finding out more.

We agreed to the consultant's plan, and on 1 June Richard was admitted to his second London hospital in a children's ward embracing a corridor of glass-sided cubicles. After the brightness of our local children's ward the sight of this made our spirits fall. The cubicle smelled strongly of disinfectant, but on close inspection was seen not to be clean. Our 'view', a drab building, was always with us, unfortunately the blind was broken. The only two bathrooms were in the next corridor, shared with the rest of the ward. I could not believe it. My son, in common with other haematology patients, was likely to have low immunity, and yet they were forced to come into close contact with other patients and parents in order to use the bathroom. What had I done, allowing Richard to come here? I had repeatedly been told over the past months, by doctors, how important it was to keep Richard free from infection.

The consultant had told me I would be able to stay with Richard but, foolishly perhaps, I had not expected to have to sleep on the floor, and was therefore ill-prepared. When bedtime arrived on our first night the only 'mattress' available was an inch-thick piece of foam. I would have taken a sleeping bag if I had realized, especially since the only way to lie flat in the tiny room was to place one's legs between those of the ancient but commodious wash-basin. The second night a mattress was obtained earlier—and it was thicker!

Despite all, Richard and I joked about our awful conditions and kept ourselves in good spirits. There were many others in the same position and it was the doctors and nurses who really mattered; they were the experts who would cure Richard. We found the nurses full of fun, from sister down to the students. The doctors always had time to speak to Richard, and he soon had his favourites.

The worst part of that treatment was the insertion of the long line in his arm under local anaesthetic. My dear little boy was so brave, saying poems and nursery rhymes whilst the doctor tried twice to place it. He began to cry silent tears, but never once making a noise. The doctor became annoyed and left the room. He had probably had a hard day and it was best to give it a rest before trying again, this time successfully. I was rather peeved the following day when Richard had a bone-marrow test under general anaesthetic. Had it not occurred to anyone that it would have been kinder to this 8-year-old child to have put the long line in then? The purpose of it was to carry the drugs; which treatment had not yet begun.

Richard was discharged after three weeks to await results. We had long ago booked a holiday in Pembrokeshire, and thanks to our local consultant's tremendous effort and the kindly co-operation of a Welsh hospital, we were able to go, promising to take Richard for a platelet transfusion three times each week. We were all so happy, because we did not know.

On our return Richard attended the hospital in London for tests, which looked well. At the beginning of the autumn term he was allowed to attend part-time school, and in new uniform a very cheerful little boy was once more amongst his friends.

A few weeks later our peace was devastated as Richard developed a non-A non-B hepatitis virus,* probably, we were told, contracted from a blood transfusion. After that nothing went right again. By the end of October, Richard had been re-admitted to hospital for a second course of drug treatment because in some cases that proved successful. Again I asked if delaying the transplant and introducing more antibodies by constant transfusions could prove detrimental, but a direct answer was not forthcoming.

Two cardiac babies died during our stay. I found it difficult to answer Richard. 'Why does God want babies in heaven, Mummy?'

Again we were home, and for a few short weeks life was sweet. Richard had his ninth birthday on 7 December and was fairly bursting with pride when, four days later, despite having been absent for most of the term, he had learned the percussion part well enough to play in the school concert. Who would have known he was ill, standing there in his newly knitted school jumper?

Two days later he bled so much I thought he was haemorrhaging. This was the slide downhill on a very slippery slope. Richard found himself back amongst his friends in our local hospital where it was discovered his liver function tests were not good. Our marvellous consultant would not let the second London hospital have Richard back before Christmas. She could cope—and she did. We attended the hospital on Christmas Eve for transfusions, returning home with instructions to telephone her at home on Christmas Day if anything was amiss. Nothing was, and consequently we all enjoyed the day at home, with Richard as full of fun and energy as any child of 9. Unless he uncovered his arms, pitted with needle marks, you could not detect he was ill. Each of those marks told a story. Richard never caused a fuss or cried over the daily needles. Our

* Hepatitis virus: This is a virus affecting the liver.

consultant used to say he could teach some of her adult patients a lesson.

In driving snow, on 12 January 1987, we travelled across the Cotswolds for what we believed would be Richard's miracle cure. Richard and I found ourselves back in a very restricted world where he was not to mix with other patients. A different consultant was now in charge, and she told me Richard's chances of surviving were somewhat less than the 70 per cent they usually reckon for transplant patients, because he made antibodies easily and his liver was still very suspect. I asked if it was really necessary—could we not have gone on with the transfusions? No. Again I tried to find out if the transfusions in the past had introduced harmful antibodies, but the subject was talked around.

Weeks went by, with endless tests, some painful and uncomfortable. Our hopes were raised by talk of new cures from abroad. All the time the doctors were trying everything in their power to avoid a transplant because Richard's liver was not thought to be in a stable enough condition for one. I was confused and worried. Richard often asked if he could go home. He would look around our 'cell' and say we were the prisoners, not those people in the high security prison next door. We felt an affinity with the prisoners, who we knew were not all bad because they periodically spent their hard-earned money on big boxes of assorted sweets for the children. We kept our spirits buoyant by reading comic verse and weird tales, helped by visits from kind friends and relations. A day did not pass without Richard receiving a card.

At this time the food was really becoming inedible. One day, supper was so appalling that sister sent for the Catering Manager, and she asked if I, too, would speak to him on behalf of the parents. Days later I found a cockroach walking across the kitchen floor. Feeling quite nauseated I ran to the bathroom, but soon regained my composure, acting somewhat out of character by causing such an enormous fuss that the whole ward was sprayed in less than two hours. Two days later a cockroach walked past my floor-space early one morning just as I awoke. The 'specimen' was posted to 10 Downing Street with a letter describing the conditions at this hospital.

Night-time was always the worst, but there was one I will never forget. Richard had spent many happy hours playing with an 11-month-old baby called Claire in the adjacent cubicle. He used to talk to her through the glass. The night she died we were very much awake, as Richard was having a transfusion which for some strange reason was always given at night. We knew Claire's heart condition had deteriorated, because she had been moved to the special nursery. The most awful scream suddenly pierced the silence. It was Claire's mother, and we knew what it meant. Richard and I were devastated.

Whilst I knew everyone at this London hospital was doing their best, I had been given so much contradictory information over the weeks I felt we needed an opinion from someone completely different.

The day we went to our fourth hospital, Richard was in excellent spirits, especially when he saw the cheerful waiting-room full of toys, and, after the consultation, the Aladdin's cave called a play-room. He did not want to return to the previous hospital and asked if he could be treated there. It was a children's hospital and he should have been treated at such an institution—but there was nothing I could do.

My head was throbbing as I walked back to the hospital car. Why hadn't I insisted on another opinion earlier? What damage had been done by this further delay? I had just been told that a letter would be written to the referring hospital, in the strongest terms, urging an early transplant. They felt it most detrimental to our son's condition to delay.

Two days later when our consultant saw Richard on the ward round I expected her to mention our visit, but she simply said that Richard should continue drug treatment for another two or three weeks, and if there was no success he would have a transplant when a bed was available. I could have cried, and so could poor Richard. Later, I asked for an appointment to see the consultant, but it was four days before my request was granted. I told her how I felt about my son's prolonged confinement in hospital, and that evening, during the ward round, we were told Richard could be transferred to our local hospital the following morning, provided we could transport him there. Tony would have moved heaven and earth to do so!

We left with the knowledge that Richard would return in a few weeks for a transplant, as soon as a bed was available.

What a welcome awaited Richard! The thoughtful staff, some of whom had visited us in London, had decorated the room and a poster with the words 'Welcome back Richard' was strewn across his bed. To get into the room he had to cut a tape. He was thrilled to be treated as a VIP and so glad to be back amongst old friends in comfortable surroundings. After ten weeks of sleeping on the floor the bed provided for me that night, beside Richard, was sheer luxury.

Two days later our inimitable local consultant told us we could go home. It was 20 March.

My darling, if only we had known, we would have done so much more in those precious few weeks you were at home; but then I suppose we would have aroused your suspicions. After all you had been through your perception was far sharper than the average 9-year-old. It was so wonderful to be with Daddy and Becca again. Friends from school visited and we walked to see new lambs and the spring flowers, fitting in, often daily, essential visits to the local hospital for transfusions.

At the beginning of April the hospital in London directing Richard's care began to make excuses for not re-admitting him. These were quite genuine, as rooms in the transplant ward had been closed owing to staff shortages. Only half of their ten rooms were open, and one of those was occupied by a fee-paying patient from abroad. How could I begrudge anyone the right to buy life?—but selfishly all I could think of was Richard. I did not care about their problems; my son was deteriorating before my eyes. Richard's platelet count was often 1 or 2 when I took him for transfusions, the slightest knock resulting in an ugly bruise.

I became weary of constant excuses and gave 'Richard's story' to a local journalist who contacted the DHSS for an explanation. Photographs were taken and, much as we hated it, Richard's picture was going to be on the front page of local and regional newspapers. Several national newspapers also contacted me. The day before the story was to be printed we were at our local hospital for a platelet transfusion when the hospital in London telephoned with a request that I take Richard in that afternoon. I was angry to have such short notice and at their very obvious reason for suddenly finding a bed! They agreed to Richard's admittance the following morning.

I am so glad now of my action, because I regard that afternoon as Richard's last in the natural world. I took him with his two dearest friends to a nearby field where they all happily played in the stream, building bridges and dams. It was a beautiful sunny day, and as the field was full of Lady's Smock flowers there were Orange Tip butterflies everywhere. This is the vision of Richard I try to have when I am down. I will not let my mind stray to his last day in hospital. Richard's last day on earth was spent in the countryside he loved.

On 29 April 1987, the electric doors of the transplant ward closed behind us, leaving me with a feeling of dread.

We were shown into a pleasant modern room with *en suite* bathroom—but it was so dark, the darkest room in the ward as I later found out, requiring electric lighting all day. I assume there was a good reason for this room being selected, but how I wish I could have seen the sky! The only section of clear glass in the window was so dirty you could barely see the brick wall four feet away. Richard was bitterly disappointed. We had been told how nice the transplant ward was in comparison with the children's ward. At least the room was large enough to walk round and I could have a camp bed.

Of all the pre-transplant treatment I found radiation the worst to witness, and I believe Richard found it the worst to endure. Something you cannot see, smell, or feel seems evil.

A doctor told me that Richard had received so many transfusions his body was full of antibodies which would fight the graft. The only way to destroy them was irradiation. At long last someone had given me a straight answer. When the professor had first seen Richard no mention had been made of radiation treatment, only chemotherapy. On the other hand, the consultant at this hospital had said only chemotherapy would be necessary. Richard was going to suffer additional pain because of the delay.

After being correctly positioned, Richard lay naked on the table with the huge arm of the radiation machine suspended above his body. His only companion was SuperTed—impervious to everything, even radiation! I could watch on a small monitor and speak on the intercom. I read Winnie the Pooh stories or spoke of Super-Ted's imaginary antics. He co-operated at all times because it was for his own good—I had told him so and he believed me. What a tremendous responsibility parents have, what trust and devotion; but do we all deserve it?

Richard had been well-prepared for the effects, both of radiation and chemotherapy treatments, and kept in good spirits throughout, despite the awful sickness. His attitude was that at last he was 'getting on with it'. He said the transplant would make him better and he would play cricket next year.

One evening I saw a nurse packing boxes in Mary's room. Richard and I had spoken at length to her parents, who told us she was in intensive care after a second transplant for aplastic anaemia, the first graft from her brother having failed. This news I found alarming, not realizing a second transplant would be necessary or even, indeed, possible. It suddenly hit me—Mary was dead. She was only 25. For the first time I began to have serious doubts about our situation.

Richard's movements were now very restricted. He was not allowed to leave his room, and I had to spend days in a long green gown. He said I looked funny, and took endless photographs with his new camera of me and every possible angle of the room.

Richard told me that the worst thing was that Rebecca was not allowed to visit him. She was not even permitted to see Richard through the glass partition fronting the corridor. We cleaned the small clear pane of glass with paper towels, enabling Rebecca, if she stood on a drainpipe, to peer in. We could not, of course, hear her because of the double glazing. The hospital rules, I was told, stated that no one under the age of 14 could go into the unit. Rebecca was not quite 12. Our children had always been very close and we found it heart-rending to watch them gazing at each other.

On Friday, 15 May, Richard had his first transplant. He was very bright during the three hours it took to transfuse Rebecca's marrow, sitting up in bed, playing games and even recording a message to his class at school.

Rebecca was the unsung hero of the day. She was not used to

hospitals. At the age of 11 she had spent months coping alone, with no one at home when she returned from school. I wondered what was going on in her mind. We had not told her too much for fear of alarming her, but was she afraid of the unknown? How I loved her, as she lay on the bed gradually coming round from the anaesthetic. I knew she had been neglected by me but hoped she would understand one day.

We now had to wait for the marrow to grow. To pass the time and take his mind away from the painful side-effects Richard set about earning some Cub badges. Tracking proved to be great fun, improvising hospital artefacts for woodland debris. The room became a forest, a field, a raging torrent. He drew an elaborate plan of an island and we imagined we were on it.

A week after transplant, Richard's lovely thick, dark hair began to fall out. He could not bear me to cut it, but I was allowed to shampoo it off. He insisted on keeping some in a polythene bag and I still have it. I found him most endearing without hair and used to kiss his head as if he was a baby once more. How he loved me and clung to me then—but, of course, there was no one else.

Tony brought Rebecca to wave at the window *en route* for home after a week of convalescence with loving grandparents. Richard so much wanted to see her properly, to touch her, but instead he wrote thanking her for her bone marrow. It was painful for Tony to leave us but we both agreed Rebecca must lead as normal a life as possible.

On 2 June my worst fears were endorsed. The doctors had not been very forthcoming of late, and it was now confirmed that the transplant had failed. Richard's was the worst case of antibodies the consultant had ever seen.

That night I could not sleep. I would will Richard to live, and that through me he would find inner strength. I fervently prayed to be given strength.

A second transplant was to be attempted. Eight had previously taken place at this hospital with five successes. As agreed, I told Richard he needed a top-up of bone marrow. Our brave son simply said, 'What about Becca, it will be worse for her?' He was so unselfish; he deserved to live. When Rebecca arrived I asked Sister if there was somewhere, a waiting room, I could go with her. There was, it appeared, nowhere in the hospital at my disposal. I took her out to lunch, but people were around us and I could not say the words. Eventually I told her on the bus, the poor child crying 'Mummy, it was so awful'. I repeated that she was the only person in the world who was a perfect match for Richard. I loved her so much, how I wished I could have been a donor. The transplant would take place on her birthday and in the middle of exams. It could not have been worse, but by the time we alighted from the bus she was happy, composed, and of course willing to help Richard 'because I love him'.

I tried to teach Richard during his illness. About this time, we spoke of Charles Darwin and evolution. He became angry and asked me if I was going to tell him there was no God. He told me that if I was, I was wrong, and he did not believe me.

Richard now faced a second course of treatment, with total body irradiation this time. On the first day of treatment Rebecca was due in out-patients, so we cunningly arranged for her to run alongside Richard's wheelchair as he was speedily pushed, masked and gowned, to Radiotherapy. They held hands through the green gown and as the radiologist was not ready when we arrived, she sat in the room waiting with him. They were so happy to be with each other again. If only the doctors could have seen them. Someone should look closely at all aspects of healing. I found it difficult to understand hospital rules that allowed various cleaners, a plumber, X-ray staff, agency nurses, and even the play-leader and teacher from the children's ward into the room of a patient with no immunity, but not the patient's sister!

The cycle repeated itself, and on 12 June Rebecca went into theatre again. This time it only took an hour and a half to transfuse, but there was no fuss as before, no feeling of expectancy, just fear. Rebecca felt and looked much worse.

It was not fair that this should happen on her twelfth birthday, and it was not fair that this should have happened to Richard at all, but he had not once said 'Why me?' throughout his illness.

I don't know how I survived that fortnight, but it must have been worse for Tony at home. Telephone conversations were often in clipped tones as the telephone was beside Richard's bed and I could not say what I really felt. Several times I wrote in my diary 'I need someone'. I often spoke to friends on the telephone but it was not the same as having another person there, to touch. I had never felt so alone.

During this time, a foreign patient's husband bade me farewell; his wife, who had aplastic anaemia, was dying; he would never see me again. They had four children. I couldn't bear it. Surely now Richard would live, the law of averages . . .

There was a feeling of comradeship, with relatives attending the four other patients. Three were not English, but even with their limited knowledge of the language we managed to communicate. At one time Catholics, Moslems, and members of the Greek Orthodox Church were praying for Richard. O that the world's leaders could be shut up in that ward for a month!

On the eleventh day after transplant a few white cells were evident, but two days later no one had mentioned them again. That night I could not sleep, tears came to my eyes when I tried. My heart would break if anything happened to Richard. Someone in the hospital knew the truth and had not told me. I wished I could have had access to the files to see that day's results. Three days later I was told a Swiss 'gene therapy', a colonizing factor from a human host, was to be used. Although not generally available it had been tried and tested successfully in Switzerland. I willingly signed the consent form for its use, as Richard was the first person in the country to be given it. After three days it was stopped as the doctors felt the second transplant had failed, Richard's body having rejected it outright with no real sign of growth.

Richard was recovering from the conditioning and beginning to feel much better, his morale being much boosted by a visit from the Chief Scout of the United Kingdom. He could not wait to tell fellow Cubs when they telephoned.

During the early evening of Tuesday, 7 July, the consultant told me that although they had not previously carried out a third transplant on anyone in Richard's situation, they would now like to as he was in such a good condition, mentally as well as medically. There was just 'a chance' he would survive. How could they know, when he was to be an experiment? I felt so choked, but had to return to Richard's room as if nothing had happened. Had I just been given his death sentence?

Early next morning, as I watched Richard sleep, I felt as if I was being torn to pieces. Tears were filling my eyes and, for once, I could not stop them. I remember running outside and holding my face up to the already hot sun to burn them away. I went back inside and tried telephoning people. No one was at home, until I rang the father of an ex-aplastic patient. He was to be my saviour over future weeks, but after speaking to him I needed to be alone and went to the only quiet place I knew of, the Chapel. The electric red candle continued to shine. The everlasting light. I stood there as it flickered. Richard had an everlasting light in him. At that moment I realized my will-power alone could not keep Richard alive. For months I had believed he would survive with my help. He had always been a strong-willed little boy and everyone had said how like me he was. There was some 'thing' stronger than me and I could not fight it.

When Tony arrived on Friday evening the consultant spoke to both of us. We could take Richard home now, where he would be able to live a few days without medication or transfusions, after which he would probably begin to haemorrhage. He would be dead within a week. I shouted an emphatic 'No'! The alternative was the third transplant, using an unrelated donor. Rebecca could not be used again. We had no hesitation in deciding on the latter course.

The consultant was obviously upset. She had tried everything in her power to save Richard and admitted that, as she felt emotionally involved, she had consulted a colleague for a final decision. How can anyone be a doctor and have their emotions constantly torn apart? She must have been in this same situation on other occasions. The life of the son we adored was in her hands—and so were we. What a courageous woman she was!

The following evening, whilst Tony sat with Richard, I walked for two hours on the large open area behind the hospital with the father who had been home that Wednesday morning. We talked of Richard and his own son, and he gave me back something I had very nearly lost, and that was hope. If it had slipped away from me then my strength would have gone and with it Richard's will to live. His wife had sent me a picture of a sky full of fluffy white clouds. On it was written 'Miracles do Happen' and I believe they do, because I know her son. He said that in his prayers for Richard he always saw him as a shining light, grinning at everyone. Richard was always smiling: teachers and staff at both hospitals had all commented on his happy disposition.

Suddenly the nursing staff seemed reticent about commenting on Richard's condition. I felt as if they were frightened of me, as were the junior doctors. I understand their feelings, but a situation does not disappear because it is ignored.

Our local consultant, having organized Richard's immediate return to her hospital, if all failed, promised that he would be able to return home where she would attend him with the aid of other staff.

That night I wrote in my diary: 'If Richard is to die I would like him to go home—just once. Why do my eyes feel dry of tears even in the Chapel where I can cry? Have I wept so many inside there are none left? Sometimes I think of life without Richard and a great fear grips me. It can't be true, it won't happen. I won't let it. Yet I know I can't stop it. It is out of my hands and I am powerless.'

My friend had spoken of faith healing. His own son had seen healers and, against all odds, was alive. We had nothing to lose and allowed one to see Richard. On 17 July, two days after the healer's visit, our hopes were raised by an encouraging blood test. It was a long time since the second transplant and the suggestion was his own marrow was recovering. The following day I was in good spirits because after three months the hospital rules would be waived and Rebecca would be allowed in to the ward. We knew why, but did not care. She was in. Richard really cried for the first time since he had been in that ward. He was such an adorable little boy. Rebecca held him close and kissed him. Rebecca so full of life, rosy and healthy. When I saw her with Richard, so happy, I refused to believe it could all end. Richard could not be snatched away from us after only nine years. They should not have been apart for so long. Had either of the ward sisters, who so sternly enforced the rules, ever had such a tragedy in their lives? I thought not.

At lunch that day I tried to tell Rebecca how seriously ill Richard was, but she seemed distant, as if she could not absorb it, or perhaps she did not want to.

Each night I listened to Richard's prayers which, more than ever, now brought tears to my eyes. After Rebecca left he thanked God for being able to see her and for making his marrow work a little, but asked if it could please work faster so he could go home. He always asked if God would please make everyone else in the hospital better: after which, I said my prayers for Richard in a cheerful voice without emotion. I really don't know how I managed it.

For weeks we lived in a dream, hoping the third transplant would be unnecessary. The blood film was promising most days, and I even began to let my mind wander to next year when Richard would lead a normal life. We played board games which Richard had ingeniously constructed. We were happy and loving in our own little world. He enjoyed music and often played his recorder, planning to have piano lessons 'like Becca' when he returned home. Some days the room was full of his class at school when the post brought twenty-five little letters or a tape. On one occasion the whole school individually said hello, and then sang 'Always There' just for Richard. We played it over and over again. It was important for Richard to feel he belonged, and Gorsley School never let him forget he was part of their community. His Arkela from the Cub Pack came, driven by the kindly Guide Leader. Richard was delighted to receive the badges he had earned in hospital. My faith in humanity had grown so much over the past months.

Then I heard that there might not be a next year for Richard. The blood was empty and after much consultation the third transplant was to go ahead. For a short while Richard was free of all transfusions and had the luxury of walking around without the encumbrance of a drip stand. He would sit on my lap for a 'proper cuddle'. Tony had the brilliant idea of playing indoor cricket—a plastic urine bottle and a ping-pong ball served their purpose well. Richard was so alive and happy we still found it difficult at times to believe he was seriously ill.

I almost did not want the final conditioning to start because I knew there would be no going back, never any chance of autologous recovery, the marrow would definitely have been destroyed and with it maybe Richard.

The day before the conditioning began the County Scout Commissioner visited to present Richard with the Cornwell Award for Courage. Richard was ecstatic, not only was it rarely given, but he was the only Cub in the county to receive it!

This final conditioning was by far the worst and on 21 August Richard had a third bone-marrow transplant.

Saturday, 29 August, and Richard was to live less than a week. My diary read: 'It is 7.40 a.m. and I am sitting beside Richard's bed being gently fanned. Richard is lying prostrate on the bed as he has done most of the day. Over the past three days his condition has deteriorated, with screaming bouts of earache and a sore throat. This, I am assured, is the delayed action of the chemotherapy drug and quite normal. What is abnormal is Richard's very high temperature—40.4 °C last night, and because he could not physically take paracetamol, I could only swab him with cool water to reduce the fever. The diamorphine was built up and they are saying, if necessary, it will be increased so much he will sleep all the time. At present he is just dozing and answers if I speak to him.

I spoke to the Chaplain at length this morning. He has proved a kind friend. I told him how I felt about life after death. He did help in a strange way because I asked him how he would feel in my position and when he told me, his thoughts were the same as mine.

Tony and Rebecca were here and in my absence this afternoon Richard sat up in bed and did a drawing with Tony 'because he felt better'.

I feel as if the truth of the situation is hitting me hard again but I must go on. I haven't wanted to eat much for days, but I must.

Tuesday, 1 September

Terrible night with very interrupted sleep. Richard had a fit of uncontrollable shivers and pain in his left side, so bad he cried. A doctor attributed this to a drug which was stopped. Richard, calm after 20 minutes, slept. Consultant thinks temperatures must be connected with graft as no infection evident. I too believe this. I look at Richard as he lies comatose from the effects of that awful heroin drug and think, you are fighting the biggest battle of your life and you must not win—the donor's marrow must win and take over your body, then you will win and live. I hate to see Richard in such distress but I am glad to see something happening. It is better than last time with nothing.

Wednesday, 3 September, 3.40 p.m.

Richard is lying on his back looking very grey and half dead, showing no sign of waking up about 4.00 as he has done for the past few days. He has a nasty cough and sounds chesty. Many tests today after terrible night when his temperature rose to 41 °C. I see Richard getting weaker before my eyes. Please don't let him go like Mary, Anna, or Joe, who died last week, all from aplastic anaemia. I haven't seen anyone get through who had that all destroying disease. I want him at least to recover enough to see home again. What I really want is for the marrow to grow. Oh for a miracle! I sit here hour after hour embroidering. I must do something.

At 6.30 p.m. the Consultant told me Richard was not expected to last the night. He had an extremely rare form of graft versus host disease. The graft was attacking his body in such a way as to cause his capillaries to leak. Breathing was laboured, as the lungs were filling with fluid. The only hope was a large dose of steroid, given intravenously. Of three previous cases in this position, one had lived.

I rang Tony, who broke down, but I remember speaking firmly and saying he must have the strength to drive the 100-mile or so journey safely. The Chaplain came and sat with us and we heard Richard utter the only words of retribution that ever passed his lips. Fighting for breath, he said 'It isn't fair'.

Tony arrived at 9.15 p.m. Richard was on oxygen, sitting on the edge of his bed. He insisted on reading his post although I said it could wait until tomorrow. I believe he knew. Up until midnight

the monitor appeared to be showing signs of improvement. Despite
the nurse's plea, Richard refused to lie down and sat on the edge
of the bed rigidly concentrating on his breathing. He fought like
that until the last few minutes of his life when he lay down. The
oxygen mask slipped and I foolishly replaced it. You see I never
gave up. Richard died at 1.41 a.m. on 4 September.

Whilst Tony and I sat with our dead son and the kindly
Chaplain, a nurse beckoned through the door. Richard had not
been dead half an hour. Tony had been told it was the hospital rules
that we vacate the room within an hour. Those words still echo in
my mind. Hospital rules! I had heard them so many times over the
past months and in my hour of greatest need they were still quoting
them at me. I stupidly asked where could we go as I knew we would
be needed in the morning to register the death. The nurse, who had
been attending my son since his admittance to the ward, suggested
we went home, knowing from numerous conversations with us that
it was over a hundred miles. When I feebly protested, she said there
was nowhere in the hospital we could stay, although a list of
addresses was available if she could find it. The Chaplain interrupted, insisting we stay with him.

With the Chaplain's aid and Richard still lying on the bed, we
stripped the wall of all our son's precious pictures and literally
hundreds of well-wishers' cards. It seemed almost immoral to do
this in front of Richard. I then had the task of packing my darling
son's clothes and toys. The nurse had meanwhile pointed out that
we could return in the morning to pack. I could not believe my ears.
She was a kindly girl with the best intentions but she really did not
have the slightest idea how we felt. I could never return to that
room.

Richard's story cannot end without mention of the person who
was probably dearest to him in all the world, Rebecca. Immediately
she saw me alone she knew. 'Where's Richard?' I simply told her
that something awful had happened and he was dead. She threw
her arms around me and hugged me close to her. The tears did not
come for some minutes.

Ever since she has been the greatest comfort to Tony and I, but will never mention Richard. I think she finds it too unbearably painful. I mention him, daily, but get little response. I hope one day she will feel less pain.

I wrote this story six months after Richard's death but time has not healed. That is a very ill-used phrase. The physical and mental pain is worse. I will never be the same again, because my heart is truly broken.

Despite all, I will never lose my enthusiasm for life. I have the finest example to follow: my son's. Life is worth living. Richard proved that by living more in nine years than some do in ninety. It is April and I have just returned from a walk, as Richard and I used to, marvelling at all the new life I saw around me in the fields and woods. I felt, as I often do, that Richard was with me.

RICHARD

Aplastic anaemia is a rare disorder affecting the bone marrow which decreases the production of red cells in the blood and usually also of other blood constituents to some degree. Some cases of aplastic anaemia are found in association with a recognized group of congenital problems. Most cases fall into either an acquired group (following exposure to toxic agents, some drugs or infection) or a group of unknown causes.

Some children's marrow responds to treatment with steroid or other drugs. This response may be temporary or permanent.

Bone-marrow transplantation is increasingly being used successfully in the treatment of aplastic anaemia of some types.

V.H.

10

Andrew

SUZANNE ARMOUR

When Andrew's illness was diagnosed sixteen years ago as cystic fibrosis, he was four months old and we had already become aware that this was no simple illness that an operation or a course of drugs would cure. It was for life. We would all have to learn to live with it and that has really been the sum of all that cystic fibrosis has been for us over these sixteen years—learning to live with it.

This learning process continues, and has affected every facet of our lives as a family and as individuals. There were no guide books, no real rules, no handy DIY manuals. It has been trial and experiment all the way. We've had lots of help and advice, some expert and some useful, some simple and some inspired, some useless, some hurtful; all of it well-meaning.

The real problem with cystic fibrosis is that there are so many unknown factors. No one knows what is really the cause, no one knows the cure, no one can really predict a prognosis. Uncertainty is both a curse and a blessing, but it has taught us some skill in balancing on a tightrope between hope and despair. We try to keep reminding ourselves of what we value most about life; for each of us, for all of us as a family, and especially for Andrew.

It seems, looking back, that we quickly decided as parents that what we wanted most for Andrew was that his life should be as normal as possible. In reality, it probably took us years to work that one out and even though it seems so simple and obvious when written down, it is still enormously complicated. 'His life should be as normal as possible.' What is 'normal', what is 'possible', what about our lives, his brother's life, and just how responsible are parents for their children's lives anyway, and for how long? These are not simple questions, and after sixteen years I still think we don't really know the answers.

In the early days, when we brought our sickly baby home from hospital he seemed to have an enormous big label saying 'Cystic Fibrosis' and it was hard for us to see much else. We became totally preoccupied in all the seemingly endless facets of his care and treatment to the exclusion of almost everything else.

Slowly, we returned to something like 'normal' life, helped mainly by Andrew himself. Children are so remarkably resilient and can cope with much more than we give them credit for. In spite of what has been, and continues to be, an onerous regime of physiotherapy two or three times every single day, and a routine of over twenty tablets a day plus drugs taken via inhalers and nebulizers, there are also trips to out-patients' clinics and sessions of up to fourteen days as an in-patient in hospital. In spite of all the repetitive, time-consuming aspects of his care, Andrew has a full and busy life like any 16-year-old. Last year he gained nine A-grade GCSE exams, he plays a tough game of tennis as well as enjoying all sorts of other sports. He is clever, articulate, and amusing. However, it is not all easy and there have been some bad times and more to come.

Andrew himself knows a great deal about his illness. He has learnt to accept the fact that his adolescent growth spurt is likely to be long delayed and he has been outstripped long ago by his peer group, with their big feet, great height, and breaking voices, while he still looks about twelve years old. He has learnt to accept that he probably will never have children. He has learnt to accept all the different aspects of his treatment, some of which are not very pleasant. He has to face a future of very uncertain health. Greatest of all he has had to accept his own mortality over the last few years as he watched children he has known well with CF deteriorate in health and then learnt of their deaths. None of this has been easy or exactly 'normal'.

All sorts of people have helped us in learning to live with CF. At the front-line for us has been the hospital staff. Obviously, doctors have played an enormous role, for Andrew would never have survived without them. However, we have sometimes had ambivalent feelings about the medical profession, ranging from profound gratitude, through frustration and suspicions to resentment. This has probably been more to do with our own attitudes, so typical of our society which expects so much of doctors—that they hold the key to life and death, that they can cure anything (especially our children), and that they ought to be infallible. In a condition like CF where there are so many unknowns it is very hard to play the traditional roles. The doctors will not cure our child, and this takes a long time to sink in to unconscious attitudes.

Sometimes we felt that 'the truth' was being withheld from us. The feeling that the likely course of this illness and its prognosis could be given to us in simple quantifiable terms nagged in our minds. Just how long would Andrew stay in reasonable health, just how ill would he be next week or next year, just how long would he live at all? These were questions which we skirted around, disguised, and rarely asked outright. We knew there were no real answers but somehow felt the doctors should be able to answer them. We felt if we 'really knew' we could cope better with learning to live with CF.

Over the years we have been fortunate in Andrew's consultant. Answers to our questions have been as honest as possible, with always a gentle insistence that CF has so many unpredictable and individual facets. It has taken a long time, and the introduction several years ago of an 'annual review', to learn to stop fretting over such questions. The annual review of Andrew's current state of health spells out aspects of his condition in quantifiable terms such as lung function tests, chest X-ray, growth, height, weight, etc., to give an overall picture. Sometimes it has been disturbing to look at his condition in more objective terms and note deterioration. However, the overall benefit of feeling that we 'really know' has outweighed the pain it sometimes causes.

Hospital admissions can also create very ambivalent feelings. In a condition like CF where the parents are so actively and continuously involved in their child's care and treatment over years and years, the handing over of that care to others can be pretty nerve-racking. All sorts of things can make an enormous difference to lessening the stress of it. Some degree of continuity in the staff is vital. To walk into the ward worried, tired out by sleepless nights, and be greeted by name by a known and trusted sister, nurse, or doctor can be such a relief. Sometimes, if admissions have been fairly frequent over a period of time, a feeling can develop of being part of an extended family where all sorts of people from medical and nursing staff, physiotherapists, school teachers, cleaners, lab staff, and so on, all seem to know and care about your child. It is very reassuring.

We have been fortunate, too, to have always been encouraged to spend as much time on the ward as we needed, sleeping there when Andrew was young or if very ill. Active involvement in his care and treatment has also been encouraged and this has now been extended to bringing him home from hospital and continuing to give him intravenous antibiotics myself.

The development over recent years of the role of the Cystic Fibrosis Sister has perhaps been most helpful in providing a sense of continuity when ward staff move on but has also acted as liaison between different people and has helped get a number of new ideas and techniques off the ground. She has taught me and about a dozen other parents how to administer intravenous antibiotics so that it is now possible to continue Andrew's treatment at home, rather than spending the full fourteen days as an in-patient.

This has been an important step despite some real initial anxiety on both my part and Andrew's. However sympathetic, friendly, or caring a hospital ward may manage to be, it is still a very unnatural environment for anyone, especially a child. When he was very young, I spent a lot of time with Andrew when he was in hospital, but as he grew up he felt he needed to be more independent of me and anyway, there was school to attend by day during term-time. However, frequent admission allowed Andrew to become almost 'institutionalized' at times. He would become very preoccupied with his condition, forget about his 'normal' activities, spend long sleepless nights swapping notes with other CF children and so on. All the months we had spent constructing a 'normal' approach to living would fade away and cystic fibrosis would dominate every-thing. Aspects of treatment would become emphasized and need endless analysis. They were no longer just a part of everyday life as we had tried to make them. He would be reluctant to return to school and pick up his 'normal' life again. Children, especially adolescents, can change alliances often, and he would find his best friend was now someone else's best friend. The other children did not 'understand'. He would be behind with his work and struggle to catch up.

Hospitals tend to become the whole world to those inside them, and it is hard to hang on to the outside world in spite of all the worthwhile attempts to keep it 'normal'—special adolescent rooms, greater informality, lots of comings and goings, duvets instead of hospital bed linen, and so on. Shorter admissions, made possible by home IVs have reduced this problem, as, of course, Andrew's growing maturity has done.

On the more mundane side there have been silly little things which can cause irritations. Once a day has been arranged for discharge it is important to be able to go quickly. Sometimes, for a variety of reasons like waiting for a supply of drugs to take home, we have waited hours and hours with growing impatience. This is another area the CF sister seems to have smoothed, and it is rare now.

We have been very lucky to have always felt that we were welcome to go to the hospital at any time with any worries we had with Andrew's health. His consultant ensured that we could just ring up and say we wanted to see a doctor. It has given an enormous sense of security. We even rang the consultant from France when we were on holiday and Andrew was not so well. Because of this immediate 'front-line' approach we have tended to rather bypass our GP, although I know of other CF families who rely on theirs for much help and support. We do rely heavily on our GP to write us endless long prescriptions for Andrew. Over the years we have developed a smooth system where I use a card to indicate what we need. A friendly chemist is also invaluable. Ours has been most helpful, always keeping a good supply of Andrew's regular needs and chasing up new and unusual prescriptions with speed. He has even delivered large cartons of overnight feed mixtures to my doorstep.

Keeping track of all Andrew's different medications is quite a big job, and I still do the ordering of repeat prescriptions myself.

Andrew has managed all his pill and potion-taking himself for some years now. At first I checked carefully to make sure he had taken the right ones at the right times, but this is no longer necessary. It has been an important step towards taking more control for himself and his health. So many people organize so much of his life for him that it is important to have some independence and responsibility. It is sometimes hard for me, after all these years, to hand responsibility over to Andrew like this, but we are doing it one small step at a time. It is not very different to allowing a 'normal' teenager greater independence and self management.

Physiotherapy has been a major part of our lives for the past sixteen years and physiotherapists have also helped us. For the first three years I did all Andrew's physio on my own and exhausted both myself and him. Still stunned from the diagnosis and months of anxiety about him, I did his physio three times a day with a sort of religious fervour. No baby or toddler really enjoys being tipped over a knee or a wedge of foam and being banged. I would cajole, sing, recite nursery rhymes, talk, plead, and insist that it was a very important and serious business. Then when Andrew was about 3, a helpful physio enquired why his father didn't do his physio, too. Edward took over, and quite suddenly it all became very much more relaxed. He didn't mind if there were interruptions and diversions. He just got on with it, and he and Andrew learned to talk to each other.

As he got older, we found for some years that he could manage with physio twice a day, so morning and evening Andrew and Edward would have nearly 30 minutes together, and shared all sorts of thoughts and ideas as fathers and sons ought to do and rarely find time for. They became as thick as thieves! Meantime, I was relieved from what had become a never-ending burdensome chore. Edward and Andrew have done physio together in cars and vans, airports, hotels, tents, and gardens, but mostly in the sitting-room, where they are not isolated from the rest of the household and where they can watch TV if they want.

Andrew's older brother was reluctant for a long time to get involved, but now at 18, he is a competent and usually willing stand-in if Edward is late or away.

A degree of independence came for Andrew when a helpful doctor introduced a PEP* mask. This enabled Andrew to do his own physio, which he now does at school each lunch-time, and also enabled him to go away with the school for a few days without mother coming along, too. We don't rely on the PEP mask, but it does permit some flexibility and allows Andrew occasional changes from our traditional methods, as well as ensuring he has physio at school without making demands on other people.

Attempts to encourage Andrew in self-physiotherapy methods with controlled breathing have not been madly successful so far. We all feel 'safer' doing the physio for him, and he finds it tiring and lonely to do it by himself all the time. This will be something we have to work on for the future so that he can have greater independence.

Ignorance about CF is still pretty widespread, and sixteen years ago our own was profound. This has improved over recent years with the growing publicity given to the condition. Sometimes breakthrough ideas in research have reached the national news. I remember one miserable evening a few years ago when the TV headlines announced a breakthrough in understanding the genetic basis of CF. It seemed to imply that a cure was just around the corner. Andrew leapt up and down with excitement. The full report was more factual, explaining that although the advances in understanding were indeed dramatic, there was no cure in sight. Andrew wept. Again, our consultant has helped us understand something of the significance of the research, but also prevented us from being falsely optimistic.

We understand how important research is in this condition and have always been willing for Andrew to take part in what has felt like the 57 varieties of research projects over the years. Our willingness was always in direct proportion to the explanations that were given. We felt we needed to know each time exactly what was involved for Andrew, or for us, and any possible side-effects, be it as simple as getting tired, or waiting around for hours, or the more dramatic possibility of an adverse reaction to a drug. Taking part in some of these projects has helped us to understand CF better, too.

* see glossary.

Giving explanations that we really understand seems to be a key to the relationships between doctors and families with CF. We have usually found that the more senior the doctor, the more time and care has been spent on the explanations.

Sometimes complete changes in approach have had to be explained, as in the case of dietary advice. When Andrew was young, CF children were recommended low fat, high protein diets, and I spent years training the whole family to eat this way. Chocolate didn't appear in the house, we never had chips or whipped cream. We consoled ourselves that it was a healthy diet and better for all of us. Then some years ago, with the introduction of much improved replacement enzymes, we found Andrew being recommended a high calorie diet with plenty of fat. It was hard to change ingrained ideas and he still can't eat whipped cream without feeling nauseated, but the chocolate was no problem! We still never have chips, and I rarely use a frying pan, but this is now for the rest of the family's health and not Andrew.

Poor nourishment can be a problem for many CF children in spite of adequate calorie and protein intakes. This affects their growth and development and has been an increasing problem for Andrew. He just couldn't eat the quantity of food needed to keep his calorie intake the 1 ½ times of what would be normal, and that he really needed. The introduction of overnight feeding with a high protein/calorie mixture via a naso-gastric tube has improved his nutrition, his energy, and hence his level of activity, and his overall health. At first, the idea of passing a tube via the nose into his stomach five nights a week and linking himself up to a pump didn't appeal very much, but he was willing to give it a trial. After several weeks he began to notice an improvement in how he felt, and his weight increased. He willingly continues his treatment now and notices if he misses it when away for the night. Perhaps one of the greatest advantages for the family has been the reduction in tension over mealtimes, when one teenager wolfed everything in sight while the other sat pushing the food around his plate while diverting attention from his failure to eat with all the cunning of an expert. Now his appetite is actually improving and he eats what he feels he can cope with and I no longer fuss and fret about it.

Many of our family and friends have provided unfailing interest and support for us in our living with CF. There were some in the early days in particular, who helped us come to terms with CF and didn't flinch from our pain and misery. Others found they couldn't cope with it, and we quickly learned to differentiate between those who really did want to know, and those who were merely being polite when they asked after Andrew. We learnt to tell the latter that 'He was fine', and quickly pass on to other things. Sometimes we would get it wrong and be hurt by their lack of understanding, as when someone would say 'Oh well never mind, he will grow out of it as he gets older'.

Just what to tell people in explanation about Andrew's condition can sometimes be very difficult, especially if they know nothing about CF. As Andrew has grown older, I now leave this more and more to him. Sometimes he feels like explaining in full, and at others he glosses over the problems by saying he has chest problems, 'a bit like asthma'. A recent week spent on work experience was a case in point. Knowing he was unlikely to have any contact with the same people in the future he was reluctant to tell them. He wanted no sympathy, no special treatment. He wanted to be normal! This created its own difficulties as he struggled to avoid proximity to chain-smokers and to keep out of very dusty situations. He struggled through the week and finished it exhausted but exultant. He had done it all on his own terms and grew considerably in self-confidence as a result. Longer-term situations do require adequate explanations for everyone's sake, but these can be limited to only those matters which concern that particular situation.

Schooling was little problem in the local small infant and junior schools Andrew attended. A preliminary discussion with the head-teacher and then a chat each year with the new classroom teacher smoothed the way with explanations that his cough was not infectious, that he sometimes needed to go to the toilet in a hurry, and that it was important for him not to get too cold, or tired, and so on. His health was reasonable and he was much the same size as his peer group. All his treatment, drugs, etc., could be dealt with at home and there were no problems.

Secondary school opened up all sorts of difficulties. It had dozens of teachers, nearly a thousand children, and was a bus journey away from home—which meant Andrew no longer came home at lunch time. It was big and bustling, and Andrew had to move up and down stairs carrying a bag of books from classroom to classroom. It was all a bit much and in spite of my preliminary chats with the headmaster, year head, and form tutor, Andrew had problems coping. His health deteriorated and he spent nearly a term of that first year altogether in hospital. We began to wonder how he could cope and when someone mentioned the possibility of special schooling if things went on getting worse, we were appalled. This was not the 'normal' life we had hoped for Andrew.

After a couple of sessions with his form tutor, who went out of her way to be helpful, we worked out several new strategies to help Andrew cope. He was given free access to a staff office where he could use his PEP mask over a foam wedge in privacy at lunchtime. He was allowed to leave classes early without having to explain each time, so that his lunch-break was not cut too short. All the staff knew that Andrew could stay indoors whenever he felt like it without having to explain that it was too cold, or too hot, or he was just too tired. He chose himself whether or not to do PE, and has never used his illness to get out of things. A team of classmates carried his bag around for him if, and when, he wanted them to. He had a couple of half-days off a week for some months whenever he felt very tired.

We also arranged for the local authority to provide him with transport to and from school in a taxi, which shortened his day for him and saved him from standing in the rain, etc., at the bus stop. He still has to get up pretty early for his physio, nebulizers, and so on to be fitted in with all the other early-morning things, like breakfast! Together with several hospital admissions this new regime seemed to pull Andrew back up again. Now he negotiates most of these arrangements for himself if and when he needs them, and the staff continue to be caring and flexible. Most of them seem to admire Andrew for his active and enthusiastic participation in all aspects of school life and respect his judgements about his needs or limitations. Naturally, some of the children resented his seeming freedom to come and go as he pleases, but a quiet chat with his form-mates by the form tutor that first year explained some of his problems to them and they have been remarkably tolerant and caring. As they have continued to outstrip him in their growth and development they have continued to treat him in just the same old way. He doesn't want sympathy, or special treatment, and especially not pity. He has managed, mainly by being exceptionally articulate, to hold his own.

Looking about 12 years old when you are really a very bright 16-year-old who has a great deal of maturity, can pose all sorts of problems, from not being allowed into '15' movies, or to take books out of the adult section of the library, to having people call him 'sweet' and patting him on the head. He mostly takes it in good grace, understanding that the mistake is easy to make and that they mean well. It takes a great deal of self-confidence to challenge people who patronize him, and he usually lets it pass.

One of the great assets we have had in helping Andrew lead a normal life was the great good fortune that he has an older, healthy brother. He has treated Andrew as perfectly 'normal' since he was a baby—a normal younger brother to befriend, boss about, or boast to, and they are the best of friends, too. This has been of immeasurably benefit to Andrew and has provided him with a 'normal' role-model for growing up. It has also stopped him being the sole focus of parental attention, and anxiety. It has prevented him from being totally spoilt and helped to keep a sense of normality about much of our family life.

The CF Trust has provided a useful link for many CF families and is a source of useful leaflets and a news magazine. We have also got to know quite a large number of CF families, especially those whose children have been in hospital at the same time as Andrew. Here again we have had a somewhat ambivalent approach. There is no one in the world who quite 'understands' like another CF parent, all about what living with CF means. However, we have been reluctant to get too close because often this would mean too great an emphasis on CF and make it more difficult to keep it just a part of our lives, and not the centre.

We have watched the other children we know with CF, growing up and coping in their different ways. Some we have had to see deteriorate in health, and we have had to learn to accept the deaths of some. This has been very hard sometimes, and we have rationalized it as best we could and talked about it as much as we could bear, and sometimes wept about them—sometimes for them, and sometimes for us. I don't know if this is something we will have to face in the near or distant future and it frightens us all. However, we feel that as long as the quality of Andrew's life can be kept as full and rich as possible, every single day of his life is of value. When I have been morbid about it sometimes, my husband has reminded me of our resolve long ago to make his life as normal as possible. Normal children don't have their lives spoilt by worrying about events in the future.

ANDREW

Cystic fibrosis (CF) is the commonest severe genetic disorder in Caucasians, affecting 1 in 2000 of the population. One in 20 of the population carry a single CF gene. A child who receives this gene from both parents will suffer from the disease.

Individuals with cystic fibrosis have respiratory (chest) and digestive problems. Treatment always includes a demanding daily regime of physiotherapy for the chest, and complex medication. Digestive enzymes, which are needed to break down food which has been eaten, are decreased in cystic fibrosis and need to be taken as medication. Long-term chest problems may cause deterioration in health and, later, strain on the heart. People with cystic fibrosis are increasingly living longer but, as yet, there is no known cure.

V.H.

11

Hamish

ANTONYA and ALASTAIR COOPER

Antonya

At the beginning of 1980, our son Hamish was outwardly a healthy energetic and fun loving boy of 5. By his sixth birthday in February of that year, though still appearing well, he had occasionally complained of slight abdominal pain. We all know that often crops up with young children. I was not unduly concerned, though I discreetly checked for worries at school and sometimes took more interest in his stools. During the following weeks the tummy aches were more frequently mentioned and his normally voracious appetite slackened off. Inside me alarm bells started ringing. Early in May I began what was to prove a long and agonizing series of visits to our local Health Centre.

Our own doctor was away on sabbatical. As a family we had not attended our Health Centre much until then. He was certainly the only member of the practice who really *knew* Hamish. Only he could have seen for himself that in comparison with the child's usual appearance he was indeed not well. The colour was fading from his face, the robust body becoming thinner and more lethargic. Pain was sometimes in his thigh sometimes in his chest and his abdomen. Daily it presented in different places. My son's sparkle was disappearing. Friends and teachers commented.

During the course of 13 weeks we consulted five different GPs (none of them our own doctor, who was still away), and a sixth GP on the phone when Hamish ran a particularly high fever in the middle of one night. None of them, while listening most sympathetically, could provide a firm diagnosis. I was told repeatedly that it was probably a 'virus' and it should eventually go away. I requested a haemoglobin* count. While revealing slight anaemia it was not considered significant.

At the beginning of July I could stand it no longer. Something inside me knew my son was very seriously ill. With no forthcoming referral from any GP we made a private appointment with a local consultant paediatrician. The night before, I wrote down every detail of the case history to that time. Hamish was examined at great length. I was gently told no problem could be found. The fear I felt at that point was almost stifling. I took a deep breath and insisted on two specific tests. One, a broader spectrum blood count (in desperation I suggested testing for glandular fever), and two, a simple chest X-ray. The latter could surely not offend this paediatrician who was, quite reasonably, keen not to inflict invasive procedures on a child for no apparent reason—and incidentally, it informed me for the first time that Hamish's heart was on the right side of his chest! Within 24 hours we received a phone call. Hamish's blood ESR† was very high. We were asked to admit him immediately to the hospital for investigation.

I *know* they had a list. It went, I guess, from common cold to cancer. As each day passed and each IVP, ECG, US scan,‡ and blood sample was taken I found myself preparing my mind to cope with what I knew would come. On 16 July 1980 I was told that my son had a stage IV neuroblastoma and without treatment was likely to survive for 3–4 months. It's hard to understand, but my tears were of relief—at last someone had recognized our plight.

Where long illness is involved bereavement can start as soon as you know that death is inevitable.

Alastair

Nobody had taken Antonya as seriously as they should—me

---

* Haemoglobin: Red oxygen-carrying pigment in the blood.
† ESR: This implies the presence of inflammation or infection.
‡ IVP, ECG, US scan: X-ray and electrical tests.

included, I suppose. To that extent I had not been as supportive as I could have been—I am a man whose glass is always half full rather than half empty, and I had always thought that something would be diagnosed which was relatively easy to cure. It is, in fact, in Antonya's nature to be assertive, and by being so she curtailed not only her 'anxiety of ignorance' but also Hamish's painful symptoms. But many mothers are not willing or able to be so, and it is surely wrong that assertiveness is necessary for action to be taken. The large majority of doctors we speak to pay lip service to 'listening to mother when child is ill'. This was not our experience in practice.

I was shattered by the diagnosis of cancer, even though Antonya had been expecting something of the sort. We were offered treatment at a London hospital, although we were warned that the cure rate was very low, and the treatment extremely unpleasant. Were we right to afford him the chance of life regardless of the suffering involved? (Were we selfish to put Hamish through chemotherapy at all?) I am sure that, with many diseases, doctors can offer firm advice to parents, but this disease and its treatment was so relatively unknown that we had to rely on instinct and make an act of faith. Antonya and I did not find it easy to agree, but now we both have no doubt that we made the right decision.

The proposed treatment was six sessions of in-hospital chemotherapy, each lasting four days or so, with about three weeks in between for the blood to recover. We were advised of hair-loss and other probable side-effects. Then they would attempt a bone-marrow transplant, surgery, with slow recovery, if very lucky, all to happen over a period of a year or so. This, at least, was the theory. We had long talks with the consultant in charge, a man for whom we developed great affection as well as respect. We learned, over time, that the reason for not being precise about proposed treatment plans was not evasion, but his awareness that the human body subjected to such chemical attack does not work entirely to a pre-ordained schedule. Timing did indeed prove to be very unpredictable. Each child's blood recovers at its own speed. I am lucky to work in a family business which allows me to be absent for long and variable periods, but we know how hard it is for most families to be together at times like that. We were really on permanent standby.

Hamish's school, where Tabitha his young sister was also a pupil, was tremendously supportive. We had to strike that wonderful balance whereby (1), he could attend whenever possible (which allowed him to carry on feeling 'normal'); (2), the staff understood what was going on, without the terminal nature of his illness being subject for open discussion; and (3), that Tabitha could attend without feeling that she had an 'odd' or 'dying' brother. We both believe that his continuing school attendance was a very important 'normalizing' factor in his life, and if child patients can be helped to do just that (if necessary the GP could go and talk to the school head), it will greatly be helping patient morale.

Antonya

Our lives were now fully hospital orientated. The initial period of forming relationships with our London hospital's caring team had been tense. But not for long. Gradually it was understood that we were demanding parents on the information front. I think we must have made an alarming impact, with our hunger for every detail of clinical knowledge and our pressure fully to integrate the medical procedures.

Occasional treatments were allowed at our local hospital, though not without problems. For many medics this was a less familiar ball-game. The specialist hospital could insert intravenous cannulas with ease and practice. There were agonizing moments when the less-practised personnel were not so adept. Also, I remember acting as carrier for one of the cytotoxic drugs, cisplatin, then in trial usage. At another point, Hamish was in one hospital receiving treatment while Alastair was in another having his cartilage removed!

In February 1981, already living on borrowed time, Hamish was given a bone-marrow autograft at the hospital in London. This is a procedure whereby a sample of the patient's bone marrow is

removed, the patient is intensively treated, in the hope of eradic-
ating all disease, and the sample of bone marrow is then replaced.
During the anaesthetized period needed for the bone-marrow
'harvest' he had, inserted, a central line, a Hickmann catheter. This
was to affect our lives in many ways, not least because, by then,
Hamish had 'clocked' up 100 needles! I was taught how to service
this by scrubbing up, gloving up, removing and refreshing the
heparin 'lock' every alternate day, and occasionally taking blood
for a count. Hamish took 4 weeks, in barrier conditions, to suffer
and recover from the large dose of melphalan that it was hoped
would eradicate his bone-marrow metastases. His digestive tract
was ulcerated, from mouth to anus, and he was fed intravenously.
Still—he managed to smile. His spirit was indomitable, while our
honest information to him was unwavering. We drew on each
other's support, on the loving care of the medical staff, and not
least on the invaluable listening ear of the chief psychologist at the
hospital.

When Hamish's blood count rose again, from almost nil to
acceptable, albeit vulnerable levels, we returned home and he to
school. I was able to prevent his immunodeficient system from
exposure to frequent 'infection-riddled' hospital visits by taking
blood samples from the Hickmann catheter for screenings. Every
3 to 4 weeks he received red cell and sometimes platelet transfusions
at the local hospital, where I was a necessary part of the medical
team, being the only one familiar with the catheter. Even our consultant paediatrician seemed grateful for my party piece. Life
through that summer was being lived from day to day.

Alastair

When Hamish had sufficiently recovered from the autograft he had
to face the operation intended to remove the primary tumour.
Although this was reduced from its original size of a grapefruit, it
was still the size of a tangerine. Antonya knows—she later went to
see it in the pathology lab. Our son was almost cut in half across his
abdomen in the enormous effort to remove all that was possible.

Amazingly, he was on his bicycle at home (albeit gingerly!) immediately after his release 8 days later!

After the blood and the body had recovered from autograft and operation, the final attack was radiotherapy. This involved 15 sessions at another London hospital and was done over 3 weeks as an out-patient. One of us took him on that long journey daily. After that we had a painfully wonderful late summer. The sun shone; we went, at last, on holiday; Hamish looked well and his hair re-grew. Apart from a slight lack of stamina he looked as healthy as one could wish. Some people wondered, more or less openly, whether we had overstated the severity of his condition. He started his new school that autumn and was so proud. We knew it would not last for ever but had hoped for a longer period of remission than, in fact, we were granted.

Antonya

At half-term Hamish had his thirteenth blood transfusion! It was now becoming common for him to show allergic reaction to these, so the ensuing familiar fever was something I felt able to cope with at home. The next day we were back in hospital. During the night his right ankle had become swollen, hot, and very painful. He had septic arthritis! (an infection in a joint). This is nowadays relatively rare but in 1984 another of our children had it. She is now fully better, but what a cruel coincidence!

A week or so before that point at our London hospital, Hamish had produced a disappointing VMA* result. In this knowledge we asked that the 'orthopod' aspirating our son's ankle should also do a bone-marrow trephine. It confirmed our very worst fears; that again there were widespread metastases. Our utmost aim was to get Hamish back home for his terminal weeks. He somehow survived the rampant bacterial infection in his body and, well into a course of hefty antibiotics, and with his lower leg encased in plaster, we left hospital for the last time.

* Vanilyl mandelic acid is a marker in the blood of neuroblastoma.

Our GP had been back in business since the previous autumn. His support since then had been magnificent. He had stood alongside and listened and cared on so many occasions, way beyond the generally accepted 'call of duty'. Now he was really to be put to the test. As a team we went through those next few weeks, with the equally wonderful help and love of a young Community Paediatric Nurse (attached to the local hospital). Our ability to articulate must have helped to summon equipment and organize drugs. I agonize for those who are less assertive and certain of their needs.

We would like to think that other terminally ill children could remain in home surroundings if that is what is wanted by the families. This is only possible, however, with full and active support of the local medical team, especially in the area of effective pain control.

I was heavily pregnant, but I found physical and psychological strengths even greater than during the almost 18 months since diagnosis. We had agreed that we would not submit Hamish to yet another blood transfusion. Anaemia should now be his gentle friend. We maintained regular contact with the hospital in London including conversations with and indeed a visit from the psychologist. It was he who provided the casting vote on a matter of enormous importance to me: my conviction that Hamish should be told of the probability of his death. Two or so days before he died, I manoeuvred separate conversations with both our children that imparted that knowledge to them. Hamish reacted not with fear or horror, but as if he had just been told he should go for a walk on a very stormy day—'Mama, I'd really rather not'.

Pain control was not a huge problem. We asked for, and got, what was necessary. The Hickmann catheter was a route that I knew we could use if oral administration became impractical. We had been provided with morphine sulphate elixir on leaving hospital and further supplies were readily available at our request. Most importantly, on the one home visit from our local consultant paediatrician together with our GP, we asked for some 30 mg ampoules of diamorphine hydrochloride. These were willingly provided. We know that this is not necessarily standard practice but it was tremendously important to us. It was also a committed gesture of faith in our role as responsible and loving parents. Most of all it was our guarantee that, when time came, Hamish would die in comfort and with dignity. Hamish's last few hours were relatively peaceful. Some days before, he had discovered a small tumour under the skin on his chest himself. A day after that I felt a further 'string' of them across his abdomen. I prayed these signs of the consuming cancer would not manifest themselves to a frightening degree before his death. That evening he laughed with Tabitha at the bedtime story that his father read. During the night hours he and I had lucid conversation, though his breathing deteriorated by the hour. His pain control was now IV—his vomiting had determined that. Half an hour before he died he wanted the strengthening pain removed. We gave him 60 mg diamorphine hydrochloride. Hamish died, gently, at 2.30 in the morning on 1 December 1981.

Alastair

Practical matters help at difficult times. We had known that Hamish would die, so we busied ourselves with administrative detail even though we had already organized much before his death. We continued to 'work' together as we had during his illness. We still had Tabitha to consider—she needed, we felt, to see her brother's death in a way that would not 'spook' her for years to come. Seeing Hamish and attending the funeral were important aspects, we believe, of her own ability to cope. Antonya was heavily pregnant and actually produced Cassandra 2½ months later, and a fine, bonny, blue-eyed Hamish look-alike she was. It was extraordinary how some people thought that the arrival of a new baby would in any way fill the hole left by the death of another child. Discussions between bereaved parents bring up similar examples with startling speed.

Antonya

After our daughter was born, ten days late and only missing Hamish's birthday by two days, I experienced what I understand is now a recognized state called 'baby-pinks'. I was mostly euphoric. There was no lack of tears, not least because this particular baby was so like Hamish as a babe. She is now even more like her brother in every way. But things were going physically well. I even tried again to breast-feed, and this time succeeded where twice before I had failed. For three or so months I fielded the naïve suggestions from unthinking well-wishers that life was now surely back to normal!

Then slowly I realized it took more effort to cope. It was as if I was set on the Cresta run—at first the exhilaration was all-encompassing but gradually the crowd noises got to me and the excitement turned, first to apprehension, then to fear, and on to certainty of crashing. I was sinking; drowning in water. Alastair was there on the edge, able to reach the lifebuoy though not thinking to do so, and I was unable to cry for help. I couldn't believe that I was really losing grip; this was so uncharacteristic that neither I nor those close to me could recognize the signals. Indeed, I put superhuman effort into appearing normal. I had post-natal, or was it post-mortal depression.

Alastair

And now, a selfish note from me. Depressed wives are miserable, but husbands don't enjoy it much either! The sympathy from our GP to me was actually much appreciated, particularly when it was clear that the GP intended to work together with husband to treat what was clearly more than a temporary spell of 'feeling low'. There was no way that Antonya was going to pick up the phone, go to a public surgery, sit in the waiting room with cut fingers, coughs, and piles—to pour out her soul in 7 minutes, come out of surgery through a packed waiting room with her tear-stained cheeks to collect her prescription for—tranquillizers! She would not submit herself to that ordeal even if she was in the best of health! And I don't blame her.

Our GP came to see us at home, in the privacy of our own surroundings. We had talked together in advance. Yes, it was hard for the GP but it worked!

Antonya

I think even our GP had been lulled by my public face. Eventually there he was in our home, telling me about clinical depression, brain chemistry, and urging me to consider anti-depressants. I took some persuading. To me that smacked of admission of failure. My personal high standards had come crashing around my ears. Thank God that Peter is our GP. With his understanding, gentle but never patronizing guidance, I took those anti-depressants; I needed them for 18 months. During that time I went through my fourth pregnancy, put on 5½ stone, produced Matilda—the family hellraiser, and over the course of seemingly interminable months, lost that 5½ stone! I threw away the tablets and went on to baby number 5, Jemima, in December 1984. When again I felt that recognizable loss of grip some months later, I was prepared, and motivated myself to contact Peter for help. I chucked out the medication after 5 months. Two years ago I produced baby number 6 despite the contraceptive pill! His name is Barnaby—we are entrusted with another son.

I now see that through all those months of Hamish's illness I was running on overdrive. I was immensely needed to cherish and guide my dying son. Our wish to keep going as normal took huge strain, and coping with other peoples' fears and doubts alone required vast resources of fortitude. I felt very positive in such a negative situation. After his death there was still a pool of strength from which to draw supplies to help soften the growing recognition that life without Hamish was dreadful. The void grew, the emptiness became all-pervasive. The amputation of part of my very being was complete. The days without his laughter were agonizing. Alastair was grieving, just as intensely—but differently. I needed to talk, but very few wanted to allow that, mainly to protect their own embarrassment, pain and feelings of inadequacy. I felt completely alone.

Alastair

Men often don't talk about these things but we feel them just as much. The idea that there is a creature called 'the Parent' when a child is ill is nonsense. There are probably two parents, and the likelihood is that they are responding quite differently to the situation. A few visits and discussions at the child's home during and after the illness will certainly improve the quality of patient care, and in the long run, increase the efficiency of the treatment of the family as well.

Antonya

The years since Hamish's death have not diminished our immense sense of loss. It is now more than 8 years since he died, and I still ache with the thought of cuddling his little body and stroking his curly hair. It is now, perhaps, a little easier to bear the knowledge of this cruel removal from our lives. For families like ours the health professional's role is of the utmost importance. Their relationship with us needs to be empathetic unless it is to be destructive. Their natural sense of impotency in such a situation must be overcome to form a positive, guiding, caring friendship, even at cost to their emotions. Sharing emotion is showing you *really* care. Being alongside should supersede any feeling of clinical failure. Therapeutic medicine may be just for the living, but the dying and their families are still in life and need just as much lovingly given expertise.

HAMISH

Neuroblastoma is a malignant tumour of neural crest origin which may arise in any area containing sympathetic nervous system tissue, but is most commonly found in relation to the adrenal glands in the abdomen. Apart from brain tumours, neuroblastoma is the most common malignant solid tumour in childhood. It accounts for approximately 10 per cent of cancer in childhood.

Prognosis in neuroblastoma depends on age at diagnosis, stage of disease, and to a lesser extent, the site of the primary tumour. For example: 85 per cent of children who present at less than 1 year of age with Stage I disease are well and disease-free after three years, but only 5–10 per cent of all children with Stage IV disease at diagnosis are alive and disease-free after three years.

Despite progressively more aggressive therapy, with surgery, radiotherapy, and chemotherapy, only minor improvements in survival have been achieved so far.

Research continues in all fields.

V.H.

12

Epilogue

The really unexpected happens so seldom that few of us know how to deal with it. We all move, for most of the time, in a small circle of known possibilities to which we have learned the responses. Outside this circle lies chaos, a dark land without guidelines.

NINA BAWDEN (1974). *George Beneath a Paper Moon.*
Allen Lane, London.

Novelists are much better at expressing psychological ideas than psychologists; this quote elegantly sums up the overriding message of this book: when we encounter not just the unexpected but something quite outside our previous experience our world is overturned.

Today's parents in general believe not only that they *should* have the perfect baby, beautiful, intelligent, healthy, sensitive, and wise, but that they *will* have such a child. The reality of life, and death, is of course quite different, and the 'We shall have the perfect baby and live happily ever after' construct is actually quite fragile.

The theory underpinning this idea goes as follows:

Throughout our lives we gradually build up a psychological system which gives us a guide to everything we do. This guide provides us with information with which to make predictions about our immediate and far future. As children we learn, for example, that we can behave in certain ways with some people but not others: think of the differences in behaviour evoked in the same class by two different teachers.

The more elaborate our system of construing events before they occur the more comfortable, psychologically, we are. The first time we visit a new country we usually feel insecure, especially if we are alone, because we do not know enough of the language or customs of the place to feel that we are able to anticipate what is going to happen next. Once we have been there for a few days we begin to relax, because we know our way around in many senses of the phrase. So when, as parents, we find our child to be either so sick or disabled that we have no psychological system to guide us, the first experience is one of shock and threat. An intense shock to the psychological system is evident in every chapter of this book.

Another factor in the theory outlined above is that of the essential self: we all have a concept of the central nature of our personality. If pressed, we could all give examples of these key components of our inner selves: we are clever, or less clever, practical or dreamy, good with money or bad, and so on. These components change with time: the teenager's view of self is different from that of the same person fifty years later. They change also with circumstances and an outsize adjustment comes with parenthood. While by no means everyone welcomes this state, many have it as a goal from their teens onwards, or earlier, and for them it becomes the most compelling feature of their lives: they are parents before anything else, before they are men or women, black, white, or brown.

Along with this core view of oneself go other attributes which make up the essential self: we are caring parents, we are strict, or liberal, authoritarian, powerful, indispensable, relaxed . . . the list is virtually endless.

When a child is sick with, say, a cold or measles, our parenting skills come to the fore and our view of ourselves as a good father or mother is reinforced. When a child is born with a serious disability or when he or she develops a life-threatening illness we have to abdicate much of that parenting role, handing over responsibility to others. When a child dies we have lost not just that child but a crucial part of ourselves.

The practical implications of this theory are well illustrated in this book: parents need help to develop a new construct system that will enable them to find guide-lines to help them cope in their new dark land. These guide-lines take many forms, differing as circumstnces change, but they come in some sequence: before anything else there is a need for hard information about the child's condition: past, present, and future. Only when that knowledge has been provided, forming a foundation on which to build, can the new construct system be developed.

Parents also need to be restored to parenthood. In recent years much has been made of the need to regard parents as partners in education, and this view has been extended to some medical circles as well. Not only do parents now have unlimited access to their children in the more enlightened hospitals, they are often encouraged to look after them, especially at mealtimes and bedtime, and in some circumstances they take an active part in their treatment as well.

Hospital staff have, or should have, changed as well. The image of the so-called professional: remote, unfeeling, and superior, is counter-productive and has, in many hospitals, been replaced by a view that if we are to share in the care of children we should share as human beings. That may lead to staff sharing their emotions, and providing they do not lose control in so doing, this is all to the good. I would like to get away from the idea implicit in the remark heard from one mother, 'Dr X is not a proper doctor yet, she cried yesterday when she heard that Y had died.'

Part of the process of building a new psychological system, of making sense of the present, is reviewing the past, trying to fit certain events into a recognizable pattern.

Many of the parents writing in this book have given a sometimes agonizing account of how they had to struggle to convince their GP or, more worryingly, a consultant, that something was seriously amiss with their child. What is never mentioned at times like this is the number of times when a GP is right, when the mother *is* fussing unnecessarily. Nor is the rarity of the conditions always acknowledged: an average GP will see perhaps two or three cases of childhood cancer in a lifetime.

It is 7.30 p.m. and the doctor has been up since 6 that morning. There has been a succession of coughs and colds in the surgery as well as a few more serious complaints. There is a mountain of paperwork to attend to. Along comes a child who is normally as fit as a fiddle. She looks a bit peaky but the last 99 per cent of patients who had her history and her symptoms have got better with rest and warmth. So this one is different, but who is to tell?

Another issue, harder to discuss, is from a psychological point of view more important. One of the problems of books such as this is that they are written by a selected group of parents, those who have both an understanding of their own feelings and an ability to articulate them. There are thousands of others who are less in touch with what is going on or who are perfectly in touch but lack the skill or opportunity to write about their experiences.

Let me illustrate this with an account of my own. Catherine was a 12-year-old with leukaemia. She was a bright, lively girl who took an interest in everything around her. She had been in an oncology ward for long enough to know two or three children who had died. She had lost her hair, she was sensitive to her surroundings. One day I was chatting by her bedside. I had not called for anything in particular, I was just passing. In conversation, I asked her what helped her cope with a serious illness and she answered non-committally. Later, her mother was furious with me. 'How dare you talk about her being seriously ill—she knows she's ill, but she doesn't know it's serious.' This was nonsense: Catherine knew perfectly well that she was seriously ill, as conversation with the ward staff subsequently confirmed. She died a few weeks later, sadly not having been able to say goodbye to her parents.

What was happening here was mutual pretence. Catherine's parents pretended to her that they were not concerned about her illness because they did not want to upset her. With them Catherine also pretended not to be worried because she in turn did not want to upset them. This defence mechanism, like all defences, can be healthy, but it carries with it the danger of stifling significant communication, not just between parents and children but between children and others. It is the danger of complete blocking that is so worrying about mutual pretence, since it leaves children alone and vulnerable.

Denial is another common form of defence that is not mentioned in this book. Many of us practise denial in all sorts of ways, but an extreme example came from the parents of a 10-year-old boy who died in hospital on Christmas Day. His parents were not with him because they were too busy cooking Christmas dinner. We knew that they had no other children, no one else to cook for. We knew them quite well and were well aware that they were desperately worried, caring parents. We also recognized that it was their anxiety that made them deny that their son's illness was really more important than a roast turkey: if we are not there it will not happen, and anyway it's not happening at all.

There is one further strand that I would like to pick up: the frailties of the NHS. First, the shortage of nurses, especially in London hospitals, has been mentioned and is well-known. (There is a shortage of speech therapists, physiotherapists, psychologists, dieticians, technicians, and secretaries as well, for the same reason: they find it very hard indeed to live on the salaries that are offered.) But we should be concerned not only with salaries: what is only now coming to be publicly acknowledged is the demographic time-bomb. The pattern of the birth-rate recently means that we now have a great shortage not just of nurses but of young people in general. To maintain nursing at present levels we would need to enrol 50 per cent of all the girls with five O-levels or their equivalent in the next few years. In ten years' time, nurses will not be scarce just because they are poorly paid; they will not be there.

The final point is more overtly political. Although one or two parents mentioned costs incidental to treatment, there was no mention of the expenses of treatment itself, no acknowledgement of the fact that some (admittedly rare) injections can cost £1000 a time, or that operations can cost thousands of pounds. This is as it should be; for over forty years we have had a health service free at the point of delivery, and whatever else parents, patients, and staff may have had to worry about, the cost to the patient and the need to allow financial considerations to be paramount in decision-making by staff has not been a feature of our work. Now we have doctors constantly looking over their shoulders at financial statements. I am not arguing against everyone being aware of the real costs of procedures; I am worried that market forces will lead the next generation of GPs to resist seeking certain specialist help not because they have failed to recognize a serious condition but for financial reasons.

The parents writing in this book have much to give, not only to those who care for their children in hospitals and clinics, but also to our masters who determine the overall shape of the National Health Service.

Department of Psychological Medicine,   Richard Lansdown
The Hospital for Sick Children,
Great Ormond Street, London WC1

Glossary

The main medical diagnoses are explained at the end of individual chapters.

This glossary defines a few other words, phrases or abbreviations which may not fully be explained in the text.

antibodies Substances formed by the body in response to a foreign material, e.g. infecting bacteria or donated tissue. They help to fight infection but may cause rejection of transplanted material.

anti-depressant drugs Medicines used to treat depression.

blue baby A baby who is born with some types of heart problems appears 'blue' around the lips and fingernails due to a lack of oxygen in the blood.

bone marrow biopsy A procedure in which a sample of the blood-producing cells in the bone marrow is aspirated via a needle.

cardiologist A doctor who specializes in the care of patients with heart problems.

catheterization Refers to a cardiac catheterization, in which a fine plastic tube is passed along a blood vessel to allow the injection of a 'dye' which shows up on X-ray. The chambers of the heart are outlined by the 'dye' to look for abnormal heart structure or function.

CF Used as an abbreviation of cystic fibrosis.

cytotoxic drugs Literally, drugs which are toxic to cells. Such drugs are usually used in the treatment of cancer to destroy malignant cells. They often have side-effects caused by damage to normal body cells.

D and C   A procedure carried out under anaesthetic in which the inner lining of the womb is lifted off.

ECG   A tracing of the electrical activity of the heart muscle. Wires stuck onto the skin of the chest pick up the tracing.

EEG   A tracing of the electrical activity of the brain. The recording is taken from wires fixed to the scalp.

ESR   A blood test which indicates the presence of infection or inflammation in the body.

grommets   Tiny plastic tubes which can be inserted into the eardrum to allow abnormal fluid to drain from the ear. They are needed when abnormal fluid collects in the ear after ear infections, causing loss of hearing.

haemoglobin   The red pigment in the blood which carries oxygen.

hepatitis virus   A virus which affects the liver.

Hickman catheter   A cannula which gives direct access to a vein for administration of drugs or fluid.

Intensive Care Unit   The area of a hospital where seriously ill patients needing much complex care are looked after.

IV   Intravenous—directly into a vein.

IVP   A special X-ray involving the injection of a 'dye' which shows up the kidney on X-ray.

lumbar puncture   Involves taking a sample of the fluid around the spinal cord by inserting a needle between two bones in the lower spine.

PEP mask   A mask which produces a positive pressure to breathe against. This is useful in self administration of chest physiotherapy.

platelet   A blood constituent involved in clotting.

Special Care Baby Unit The area of a hospital where ill or premature babies are cared for.

US scan Produces a picture using ultrasound waves which may be useful in diagnosis.

VMA Vanilyl mandelic acid—a substance which is raised in the blood and urine of patients with neuroblastoma.

ventilator A machine used to 'breathe' for a patient.

Drug names used in the text.

cisplatin **melphalan** **DAT** **MAIZE**	Individual drugs, or combinations of drugs, used in the treatment of some cancer patients.
betadine	A brown, iodine-containing antiseptic used to clean the skin.
diamorphine hydrochloride	A powerful opiate based painkilling drug.